CULTURE, ENTERTAINMENT AND HEALTH PROMOTION IN AFRICA

edited by

Kimani Njogu

CULTURE, ENTERTAINMENT AND HEALTH PROMOTION IN AFRICA

Kimani Njogu

Population Communications International – Africa

Designed & Published by

Twaweza Communications Ltd.,
P.O. Box 66872 - 00800 Westlands,
Twaweza House, Parklands Road,
Mpesi Lane, Nairobi Kenya
Email: twaweza@nbnet.co.ke
Tel: 020 3752009
Fax: 020 3753941

for

Population Communications International – Africa

ISBN 9966 9743 26

The main funding for this publication was provided by the Ford Foundation office of Eastern Africa by supporting the Nairobi Soap Summit organized through Population Communications International – Africa

Printed in Kenya, East Africa

Contents

Dedication

Dedicated to Gideon Kariuki "Kiki" (1980 – 2004) taken away by a road accident at the peak of his youthful years.

Acknowledgement

This book would not have been possible without the support of many people. First, I would like to thank the Ford Foundation, Office of Eastern Africa for supporting the 2003 Africa Soap Summit on "Making Entertainment Useful" from which most of the ideas in this book were presented. The support of Dr. Tade Aina, Dr. Mary Ann Burris and Rob Burnet has seen these thoughts shared widely.

Secondly, I am indebted to the team at Twaweza Communications and Population Communications International for the commitment, devotion and shared vision. I would like to specifically thank Joyce Njoki, Catherine Gichuhi, Mary Mugo, George Wakaba, PJ Muriuki, Lucy Muriithi, John Shikuku, and the late Gideon Kariuki (Kiki) for withstanding pressure of putting the Summit together. Equally, I am grateful to the PCI staff in New York, notably David Andrews, Kate Randolph and Lillian Chege, for their support as I worked on this publication.

The participants at the June 2003 Soap Summit in Nairobi deserve a special mention. They were vibrant, innovative, and generous! Without them this book would not have been possible.

To you all, I say "Asanteni sana!"

Kimani Njogu
Nairobi, October 2004

Introduction

Media efforts are critical in health promotion and there are numerous initiatives in Africa that are using media outlets to improve the quality of life for people, in a holistic sense. Some of these initiatives address gender equity, HIV/AIDS, poverty, maternal-child health, malaria, environmental conservation, and access to food, shelter, and education. The mediums for these interventions range from spot advertisements to music videos, magazine programs, cartoon strips, folk performances, sports, and radio and television soap operas. Popular culture is being viewed as a vital way of dealing with serious issues through community involvement and participation.

This book results from discussions at the 2003 Nairobi Soap Summit, convened by Population Communications International – Africa and Twaweza Communications. The summit on *Making Entertainment Useful* brought together organizations and individuals who are making entertainment useful in promoting health. It was a celebration of the arts in all their various manifestations. The summit focused not only on issues and messages placed in communication interventions, but it also took a critical view of the aesthetic appeal of different art forms. It was an appreciation of artistic interventions, be they in the form of soap operas, music, cartoons and comics, performing theatre, folk theatre, photography or painting.

The Summit was a reflection on and celebration of cultural productions. In *Culture and Imperialism* (1993) Edward Said has perceptively delineated two aspects of culture. First, he argues, culture refers to practices in the arts, communication, and representation distinct to a significant degree from the political, economic and social realms and which exist within an aesthetic dimension. Cultural products have the ability to stimulate our emotions in a pleasurable manner. Second, culture refers to each society's granary of the best that has been thought and known; that has been experienced. It is what shapes a society in a particular way. Viewed in this light, culture is a form of identity.

In the contemporary world culture is mediated by a number of experiences both internal and external. Practices are interrogated, eradicated, revised, and promoted. Culture is Africa is in motion.

The Soap Summit was, therefore, a moment in Nairobi for us to see how culture is being mediated and re-energized in order to address issues of health.

In organizing this Summit, we aimed at giving participants the opportunity to discuss, among other things:

- Language, literature and social change
- Media and health education
- Interventions on HIV/AIDS and the role of culture
- Background for soap operas in Africa
  -Storytelling & modeling
  -Traditional and new popular cultures
  -Language and the arts
  -Culture as raw material
- Representation of sexuality in the arts
- Intergenerational communication
- Art and the making of African histories
- Urbanization and the media
- Media and gender
- Monitoring of media interventions
- Meeting Donor expectations
- Regulation of Entertainment
- Sustainability of Issue Based Entertainment

The Summit also provided an opportunity to participants to reflect on art as a creative intervention that provokes critical thinking.

The Summit brought together media practitioners, educationists, policy makers, donors, and health workers who shared and reflected on how popular culture can best be utilized for the good of society. Participants were from Botswana, Malawi, Nigeria, South Africa, Tanzania, Uganda, Zimbabwe, India and the USA. All of these countries have utilized entertainment in interventions on critical health and social issues.

The Summit examined various forms of entertainment from a number of perspectives, including culture, history, traditional and evolving values, innovations, language, visual images, and art as beauty. It considered the theoretical underpinnings of entertainment as a way of dealing with social issues, programmatic interventions on the continent and the monitoring and evaluation of programs. There were panel presentations, discussions, and performances in dance, poetry and puppetry. But why was this necessary?

Entertainment is an important way of engaging people at the emotional level in order to achieve certain goals. In the past, entertainment has not been taken seriously. It has, in fact been associated with sin, laziness, misleading the public, false consciousness, escapism and gratification through fantasy. However, it is becoming quite evident that popular culture can play a pivotal role in increasing levels of knowledge, changing attitudes and influencing behaviour change by getting communities to participate in dialogue and to act together in order to change their condition. Popular culture can ignite critical and responsible consciousness.

The invocation of the term 'useful entertainment' at the Summit was deliberate. While recognizing the critical role that entertainment plays in the need to appreciate and capture beauty and the aesthetic in art, relaxation, recreation and escape from hard work and other related engagements, many people think that there is a need to reflect on how it can be made even more beneficial to society by contributing to social change.

In the contemporary world, there is always some tension between the transfer of knowledge and information and the way such content is packaged. Occasionally, content is significantly degraded through the overt use of sex and violence to achieve higher ratings. The belief is that 'if it bleeds, it sells'. At other times, entertainment is given a back seat and viewed as insignificant. The end result is unengaged and bored audience. Considering the opportunities that entertainment genres provide, how can reasonable balance be ensured? Indeed, how can engaging styles in the presentation of socially relevant issues in a consistent and humanity-enhancing manner be facilitated? How can we grow audiences through entertaining interventions in order to influence social change?

Voice of Government

Governments can either hinder or facilitate social change programming. In situations where a government is an obstacle civil society organizations have far limited space on which to undertake their tasks. Their success will depend on their ability to creatively realize their vision without being deregistered or closed down. Ingenuity, subtlety, courage and sheer luck play a major role. Contrastively, if the government is facilitative, the link between civil society organization and communities is smoother. The government in this latter case contributes in the well-being of its citizens and will be unduly bothered by activities of organizations which work directly with communities. The democratic atmosphere made possible by tolerant and people-centred governments is key to the well-being of communities.

Within the context of entertainment-education, governments are called upon to support efforts by groups and individuals to make a difference. But how can this be done?

In order to answer this question, we present the speech by the Kenyan Minister for Health, Hon. Charity Ngilu, during the Nairobi summit.

On behalf of the Minister of Health, Hon. Charity Ngilu, the Deputy Director of Medical Services Dr. Joyce Onsongo read the opening speech and officially opened the Summit. This is what she said:

"Ladies and Gentlemen, it gives me great pleasure to be part of this important gathering in which issues of entertainment and health are being discussed. In most cases, the entertainment industry is taken for granted. Yet, it has the potential to play a critical role in addressing important social and health issues.

The most effective teaching strategy is that which involves the audience. When the audience is involved, they tend to identify with the issues at hand and may, in fact, change their attitudes and behaviour. Because entertainment captures the emotion of people, they have the potential to involve and influence. It is vital that we harness and develop the entertainment industry not only for its own sake but also for the sake of society. Involvement of target audiences can have a lasting effect if they can identify, bond and see an emotional value in the messages. Therefore, although it is critical that we impart the correct information to our target audience, it is equally important that messages be packaged in an attractive form. As we all know, a good meal might be destroyed by the style of presentation.

Communication is in fact, dialogue, involvement and participation. It requires creating cultural identity, trust, commitment and ownership. It is vital for the empowerment of peoples. I would like to encourage you to listen to the people in whose interest you design programs. By listening to them we are able to address important health and gender issues within their cultural context. Even as we try to change cultures, we should do so with respect and sensitivity.

Women and girls face huge challenges that need urgent attention. They require more political and economic empowerment in order to help gender specific issues. They require support in order to ensure the realization of their sexual and reproductive health and rights. This will stabilize populations through informed decisions and access to opportunities, not coercion and control. There are also issues of violence against women, safe motherhood, and teenage pregnancies. You will agree with me that women have an inherent right to enjoy quality health at all times.

Through your work in entertainment you have the unique ability to share information and create mutual understanding and collective action toward a common goal. You are able to facilitate social change through community dialogue and the development of social catalysts. As you know, communities do not spontaneously initiate dialogue and action. Rather, they require agents of change. Your programs can become external agents of social transformation in our communities.

In your programming, I would like to encourage you to deal with important health issues such as HIV/AIDS, malaria, tuberculosis, and basic hygiene. These are serious problems in our societies. Assist communities to recognize the problems in their midst and the importance of dealing with these individually and collectively. Knowing that a problem exists in our societies is important but insufficient; we must take the next logical step of dealing with it. Furthermore, I would advise you to identify and involve leaders and stakeholders and assist communities feel that they are capable of making a difference. Let us not impose solutions; instead let us seek to draw them from our target audience.

You will be discussing the importance of conducting research when designing issue-based entertainment programs. Research before implementation is very important. But, in my view, it ought to be continuous. Monitor and evaluate your programs so that you can improve on them and identify emerging issues in our societies.

One of the major challenges we are facing in Africa is HIV/AIDS and I have been informed that in many of your discussions you will take the time to reflect on this pandemic. In Kenya, the government has put HIV/AIDS top in its agenda. The President has appointed an HIV/AIDS Cabinet Committee, which he personally chairs. We are concerned with a wide range of issues including prevention, anti-retroviral drugs, financial resources, stigmatization, orphaned children, people living with HIV/AIDS, the place of community and religious leaders, the role of culture, the effects on women and girls and prevalence rates. We estimate that 2 million people are living with the virus in Kenya and that 200,000 may need treatment.

We face massive challenges of sustaining and expanding successes in prevention and providing adequate treatment, care and support for people living with HIV/AIDS or orphaned by the epidemic. Africa must implement a full prevention package in the next two years in order to cut the number of new infections by 29 million by 2010. The package could also help achieve the target of reducing HIV prevalence rates among young people by 25% by 2010, as set in the Declaration of Commitment on HIV/AIDS. We cannot afford any delays.

The Ministry of Health is committed to a national health insurance plan. Hopefully, this plan will cater for the treatment of opportunistic infections and full-blown AIDS. We hope that our partners can assist us in ensuring the realization of this objective. We also hope that the private sector can support us in this endeavour by expanding its reach and showing greater social responsibility."

This speech suggests a willingness of Government to work with creative people in the resolution of the critical issues facing Africa. Involving governments in the development of entertainment-education initiatives can have the effect of creating a facilitative environment as well as contributing to sustainability.

I

Notes on Reproductive Health and Soap Operas in Africa

Although the world has realized dramatic advances in health, crucial challenges still remain, especially in Africa. Health is a basic human right and is essential for social and economic development. Some of the prerequisites for health are peace, shelter, education, social security, food, the empowerment of women, social justice, and equity. It is imperative, therefore, that health related work proceeds from a broad perspective, allowing for a wide scanning of the social, political and economic terrain. As we more into the 21st century, there is a critical need to come up with intervening strategies to ensure the promotion of health for all. Of vital importance is the reaffirmation that "health is not the absence of disease." Also, it is the view that we need to target the quality of life of people more directly so that the un-freedoms (hunger, shelter, education and so on) that bedevil them may be redressed. No meaningful development can be achieved without addressing the unfreedoms of people. The unfreedoms in Africa are particularly unnerving. Let us consider the case of Kenya briefly with regard to health.

Currently the population of Kenya is estimated at 31 million, of whom 5 percent are under one year; 20 percent under five years; and 50 percent under fifteen years. Forty-five percent of adolescent women are mothers or pregnant with their first child by the age of 19, and nearly 93 percent of women between 25 and 29 years of age have given birth at least once (KDHS, 1998). The population growth rate stood at 3 percent in 1964 when Kenya achieved independence. It rose to a record 4 percent in 1979, before declining to 2.9 percent in mid-1995. According to the 2003 KDHS the total fertility rate (TFR) in Kenya stood at 5.0 in 2003. This indicates a rise in fertility rates over the last five years as there was decline in TFR from 8.1 in 1975/78 to 5.4 in 1990/93 and 4.7 in 1995/98. This also indicates that Kenya's fertility decline in the previous two decades has stagnated.

And there are other serious health problems which require urgent and consistent action. The leading causes of mortality in Kenya are related to maternal and perinatal causes; AIDS-related diseases, such as pneumonia and tuberculosis; malaria; and injury. Child mortality in 2003 KDHS was 78/1000 births while it stood at 60/1000 in 1989, 62/1000 in 1993 and 74/1000 in 1998. Thus comparing of mortality rates recorded in 2003 KDHS with the earlier surveys shows an increase in both infant and under five mortality rates from 1989 to 2003. Although the causes of the increased mortality may be numerous, the major causes of morbidity and mortality in Kenya are diseases and conditions that are preventable. We need to provide interventions that will ensure that the health hazards are erased.

Since the sexual, reproductive, and marital years of Kenyans typically start early, the need for accurate and comprehensive information as well as high-quality services begins in adolescence. Reproductive health, HIV/AIDS, gender equality, and other social and cultural issues continue to be critical for people of all ages in Africa. They must be addressed at the family, community and national levels.

It is generally recognized that issues of reproductive health are central to the emotional, social and economic well being of individuals and societies. In the case of Africa, they are unfortunately compounded by fast population growth, not in harmony with social and economic development. The immediate effects of unchecked population growth and poor reproductive health include:

♦ Poverty which leads to, among other things, poor housing; poor nutrition; land conflicts; unemployment; non-literacy; drug abuse; and street children
♦ Low status of women;
♦ Massive water shortages due to aridity, intermittent droughts, desertification, and societal stress;
♦ Migrations, especially rural-urban and rural-rural;
♦ Lack of access to quality health services;
♦ Environmental deterioration, including deforestation; soil degradation; overgrazing; watershed destruction; and urban encroachment on prime agricultural land;

Thus it is vital to address issues of fertility and reproductive health because they are life saving and also because of their other implications on the quality of life of people. Significantly, health interventions ought to be holistic in conception and implementation.

Although there has been some success in guiding people's attitudes about sexuality in Africa over the last decade, a lot still needs to be done. In the eyes of many people, the major stumbling block in these efforts is the male factor. Due to the skewed nature of the power relations in families, decisions on pregnancy are overwhelmingly made by men. And these decisions are made with very little consultation between the spouses, because communication on sexuality matters in the families is negligible. The situation is not different for adolescents. It may even be worse; yet they need information urgently and without further delay.

Young people are faced with a myriad of problems and complications as they struggle to deal with growth and identity formation, within a globalizing social and economic setup. They are in dire need of information on their own sexuality and how to deal with it and are getting conflicting signals from the mass media, as well as their immediate environment. Young people are under intense pressure from their peers to engage in premarital sex, which is in most cases unprotected. This puts them in the danger of becoming pregnant and contracting STIs, including HIV/AIDS. Indeed, the HIV/AIDS epidemic presents frightening challenges and all health programs should look for ways of dealing with it as a matter of urgency. Although many people know about the epidemic, they are not taking enough precautions to protect themselves. This is in spite of the significantly negative impact the disease has had on families through loss of loved ones, and on communities, through an increase on the burden of caring for the sick. Old people have to start bringing up children all over again. Social responsibilities are being drastically reversed; communities are in a crisis and disharmony.

Although knowledge and attitudinal levels on reproductive health are slightly high in a number of developing countries than was the case a decade ago, they do not necessarily translate into responsible behavior. This is as a challenge to social scientists and workers within the area of family health. The mass media can play an important role in changing the direction of events. Indeed, there is a strong association between exposure to mass media messages and reproductive behavior. The exposure leads to greater knowledge and use of contraception, in the future preferences for fewer children and intention to stop child bearing and to engage in responsible sex. Moreover, exposure to media is associated with delayed onset of sexual intercourse and later age at marriage. These have implications on overall health and well being of individuals and communities.

In designing effective media programs, it would be vital to depict the value of higher education and the disadvantages of lack of education. The pursuit of higher education and career goals has the effect of delaying the onset of sexual activity and child bearing and contributes in broadening of choices, especially among women. The world and operational spaces are made wider, opportunities are opened. Energies among the youth are consequently directed elsewhere. The application of the social learning theory in this matter implies that adolescents are more likely to prevent pregnancy if they *know* how to abstain or use contraceptives; if they have the *skill* to do what they know; if they *think* that they can effectively use the skill, and if they *believe* in the personal value of succeeding and self actualizing.

Adolescent Pregnancy

Many will agree that adolescent pregnancy has adverse medical, demographic, educational and socio-economic consequences. It is related to truncated educational attainment and, consequently, to lowered economic power. Inspite of the effects of teenage pregnancy, the countries of sub-Saharan Africa continue to have the highest levels of early childbearing in the world and in some countries as many as 40% of women have their first child before the age of eighteen. This situation has generally led to less access to educational and professional opportunities among females in Africa. As stated above, one of the social-economic effects of early childbearing is limited access to higher education. For instance, out of the 10,934 students who were selected to join Kenyan public universities in the 1991 / 1992 academic year only 2,542 were female and in 1995, women comprised 30% of the intake. Early child bearing is one of the factors leading to the low university admission among female students in Kenya. In addition, adolescent pregnancy has implications on reproductive health generally. It results, in many cases, from unprotected sex, which also exposes the youth to STIs and HIV/AIDS.

Maybe by creating alternative role models these challenges can be minimized. People are constantly engaged in building new images, as mental representations of stories, or through updating old models of episodes they witness, participate in, read or hear about. Models play a role in discourse production and comprehension. According to Bandura's social learning theory values may be converted into behavior by presenting appropriate individuals who practice the required behavior and are rewarded in the face of the observer. The audience's behavior is influenced because it undergoes a vicarious experience. Stories in drama may contribute to listeners identifying with the positive values advanced by characters in the episodes. *Identification*, as a process in which an individual links his or her feelings, thoughts, and action with those of another person who acts as a model, plays a key role in behavior change among adolescents. It can be anchored deliberately so that it serves individuals and communities; for instance through serial dramas.

The potential of the serial drama genre as a strategy to intervene in people's behavior patterns and practices was recognized at the 1994 International Conference on Population and Development in Cairo. In Article 11:23 it is recognized that 'there is need to make greater use of entertainment media, including radio and television soap operas and drama, folk theatre and other traditional media to encourage public discussion of important but sometimes sensitive topics". Yet most radio and television drama programs, which are not research-based and lack a transformational theory, continue to perpetuate essentialist, biologically determined female and male subject positions. But as Nochimson (1992) has convincingly argued, serial drama has the capacity to be positively transformed into a kind of feminine discourse. It has the potential of acting as a major communication channel that foregrounds female subjecthood. Although an essentialist femininity and masculinity does find expression in the genre, I am convinced that an inclusive and gender sensitive serial drama model has the potential of centralizing female subjectivity and positively influencing the educational and career ambitions of teenage women in Africa. It has the capacity to positively empower women and men psychologically and contribute in their socio-economic development.

The absence of theoretical models that would inform teenage education on their sexuality has contributed to greater alienation between adolescents and adults. Yet, by foregrounding the concept of *identification* and community dialogue and action, informed by existing social-cultural contexts, in literary creativity and service provision we may be able to engage in meaningful exchanges with teenagers and intervene in this medical, educational, and socio-economic problem. In my view, in most rural areas where early child bearing is sanctioned by culture, identification plays a role in perpetuating teenage sexual practices. But this process may be reserved through the serial drama genre by presenting alternative sites of identification for the adolescent. We know, for example, that peer influence has a profound impact on the attitudes and behavior of teenagers. This is because teenagers are prone to identifying with their peers and modeling their behavior and attitudes around other individuals with whom they interact. But how can such identification be redirected and utilized to speak more positively with teenagers? How can identification be engineered so that it can contribute to better health and well-being?

Early sexual practices among certain communities in Africa is historically linked with socio-cultural patterns which act as rites of passage to adulthood. Such patterns of life have in the past provided information circuits about issues related to family life, sexuality and so on. But most of these informational channels are disintegrating and are hardly operational. In the glare of social disintegration and rapid urbanization, early childbearing for example, has continued unchecked without the support structure of marriage or community for the teenage mother. Spatial and psychological distance between the young and the old has been broadening and efforts to introduce overt sexuality education in schools has regularly met strong opposition, clearly at times due to a confusion between sexual activity and the broader notions of sexuality and family life.

The facilitation of parent-teen communications may play a role in preventing teenage pregnancy and irresponsible sexual activity. Parents serve as role models, influence the self-esteem of their children and instill values and moral structures that may contribute positively or negatively in the development of their children. Parents practice a variety of child rearing techniques. They may, for instance, assert their power as parents to change the attitudes of their children or they may momentarily withdraw their love in order to elicit a certain behavioural pattern. Parents may also act as sources of information and feedback on sexuality. Unfortunately, that burden has been shifted over the years to teachers who are currently ill equipped to deal with it. Parents ought to start repositioning themselves and to play the role of bringing up children in more healthy atmospheres where discussions on sexuality are uninhibited.

Inspite of the immense information gap, only a few schools, churches, family planning organizations and social service agencies provide information to teenagers on their sexuality. In Kenya this information deficit was made worse by a national educational policy of expelling from schools girls who become pregnant. In contrast, school-going boys who made girls pregnant were not expelled, punished, or even counseled. Although guilty teachers are normally dismissed from the profession, government workers and politicians responsible for making girls pregnant are rarely punished. After unyielding pressure from women's movements and human rights organizations, it is now possible for a pregnant student to resume classes after delivery. But we should be putting structures in place to ensure that girls do not take part in irresponsible sex, in the first place.

In a review of adolescent sexuality among African-American teenagers, William (1991) has attempted to understand the meaning of childbearing to teenage mothers by analyzing interviews with a group of mothers who had borne two children as teenagers and another group who had borne one child during their teenage years the focus in that study is on the experiences of pregnancy and childbearing among Black adolescents in the United States and how they relate to their culture and personal circumstance. Meanwhile, in their study of teenage pregnancy in Kenya, Kiragu & Zabin (1992) recommend a multifaceted approach to adolescent sexuality behaviour. In addition, they suggest that initiatives that would increase the power of females relative to males, especially regarding sexual expectation, and those that would emphasizes male sexual accountability 'will have far-reaching benefits for today's adolescents.' Life skills training, ability to resist pressure, condom negotiations, and planned sexual activity, access to services can have lasting effects.

The poor academic achievement of many girls and girls' sense that school is irrelevant to their needs are, at least partially, attributable to the treatment they receive in educational systems. Teachers may, for example, have different expectations of students according to gender. Moreover, educational materials continue to emphasize male achievement throughout history and ignore accomplishments by women. Few professional women are foregrounded as possible role models with whom female students could identify. In the final analysis, female students are left with few options in life. When such school experiences are coupled with socio-economic deprivation in most families, parenthood may seem the most meaningful alternative to adolescent female students. But how could communication strategies be developed that facilitate the reduction of such gender stereo-typing in schools? What anticipated pay offs exist that may be used to subvert the perception of early motherhood as a viable alternative? How can the soap opera genre, for example, be used to address alternative locations for the empowerment of female students and out of school youth?

Musick (1993:64) argues that a major crisis for teenagers is identity formation and that identity is a primary motivational force for adolescents and social environment plays a major role in identity formation. This insight may provide a window through which we may be able to view the impact of peer groups and role models for teenagers. For instance, a scarcity of models in the teenagers' immediate environment exercising other life options may be sending signals that teenage child bearing is acceptable (Williams 1991:59). The child bearing may be preceded by a number of sexual encounters, experimentations and risky behaviour. It may be the culmination of sexual escapades that may result in ill health and even death. A reversal of the current trend may be achieved through introducing models as mental representations of social situations in the environment of the teenager. What would happen, therefore, if alternative peers in the form of serial drama characters were introduced into the lives of teenagers? They may bond and affect each other positively. Identity is acquired through sustained personal efforts and adolescents need a moratorium period in which different competing alternatives, roles and opportunities are made available to them. They will then sort them out, discard some, suspend and reshape others. The serial drama model provides an opportunity for the construction of alternative and competing identities with which teenagers may relate and bond.

There is no doubt that communication between adolescents and their parents on matters of sexuality is virtually non-existent. This is the case, although people recognize that it is of paramount importance that parents "talk with" their children about the process of growing up and being responsible. Where such communication exists, girls are only informed about menstruation and how to deal with it. The communication is only peripheral to the needs of the girl-child.

On being asked why parents were not talking to adolescents about sexual matters, most adults say that they feel shy and embarrassed. They do not know how to deal with the topic. "How does one start talking about sex to one's children? Let the teachers deal with it!" Some women say that girls will stop respecting their parents if they talk about sex with them. "How shall I look at her afterwards?" Image, respect and cultural prohibitions are invoked.

Yet, the younger people want information. "We would like our parents and teachers to be straight forward and tell us everything. To be free with us.... *yaani* to be point blank..." pleads one girl speaking on behalf of all others in an interview. The others support her views. "Our teachers are not free; you ask them a question and they just laugh," says a disappointed girl. They want forthrightness and access to sexuality information.

However, the girls are against parents and teachers who give very little information but keep on exaggerating the consequences of behavior. One of them said recently, "There are some parents ... ok ... they tell you the fact, and then they keep on exaggerating ... they just keep on giving threats ... so you also decide to become tough." That toughness manifests itself in sexual activity, sometimes under dangerous circumstances. Girls also assert that they would like to get information from both parents but preferred fathers because "fathers are more serious. They are strict in whatever they say. Okay, fathers will not mince their words. But mothers always like to exaggerate things...." And fathers know the behaviour of boys and can guide the girls on how to protect themselves.

In a substantial number of cases, it is evident that most adolescents consider their parents to be old fashioned. "We would like them to keep off from the choice of our intimate friends. When they see us with friends of the opposite sex, they think we are immoral. Sometimes we are just having fun, together. It does not mean anything! They do not seem to understand the dynamics of time", they affirm. They reiterate that modern youth have a "leisure aspect in relationships." Adolescent boys feel that girls should be more careful and disciplined than boys. While recognizing that they need to respect girls, the boys feel that it is easy for girls to be cheated because they are "naive." This "naivety" may result from lack of critical information and negotiation skills.

In view of the level of sexual activity among adolescents in Africa, one would expect them to take protective measures against pregnancy and HIV/AIDS. But discussions with young people indicate that they hardly protect themselves against STI/HIV/AIDS. The reasons vary from unavailability of the services to rumours and misconception associated with the various methods. Fundamentalist religious positioning make matters worse by denying youth useful sexuality information.

On being asked whether they would be comfortable preparing themselves with condoms before a sexual encounter, girls respond that when boys find them with condoms, they say they are loose, and 'available.' This scares most girls from buying condoms, even when they know they might engage in sex. Adolescent boys also say that girls will assume they are immoral if they suggest that they use a condom during a sexual encounter. Consequently, they prefer not using condoms in order to maintain their relationship. Instead, they use condoms with prostitutes. There are also rumors about condoms. These include: (i) sex is not enjoyable if one uses a condom; (ii) the condom may come off; it can remain in the vagina and damage the uterus; (iii) condoms may burst; (iv) condoms have tiny holes and, therefore, are not really protective; (v) condoms are laced with AIDS virus to reduce the number of Africans in the world. The promotion of condoms in Africa is hence seen as part of a wider Western conspiracy; (vi) some condoms were first used in

Western countries and are sent to Africa, after being recycled. They spread disease. Africa does not trust the West.

Then there is lack of trust between boys and girls. Most boys suspect some hidden motive in their relationship with girls. In many cases, they think girls want money and gifts from them and not just friendship. They say: "If a girl approaches a boy, it cannot be because of love! Never! Girls are always scheming. They will come because the boy has something the girl wants, for example, money or education. She wants security for herself in future." In order to overcome the rumors and the problems the youth are encountering, adolescents suggest that there is need to put in place education programs that target them with messages on being responsible, communicating with parents, STIs, HIV/AIDS, reproductive health and related subjects.

Of critical importance in certain parts of Africa is the perception that girls are expected to start having sex after undergoing a cultural rite such as circumcision. Let me illustrate this, with evidence from one region. Female circumcision is high in Kisii district of Kenya and over 75% of Kisii girls are operated on reaching puberty. The operation, as a rite of passage, is accompanied by certain sexual freedom. There is the view among men that such girls are ready to start child bearing. Due to the unavailability of reproductive health services for the youth and considering the cultural value placed on marriage, among many communities in Kenya, it would appear that the practice of multiple sexual partners and teenage child bearing will continue unless these issues are addressed urgently. Education achievement is blurred by socio-cultural expectations. In fact, adolescents who place more value on education may be less vulnerable to early sexual activity and motherhood because they are more interested in pleasing their parents, other family members, and teachers through academic performance. They may also have other goals beyond gratification resulting from a relationship encounter. Consequently education seems to be an important motivator to guide fertility and sexual behaviour in the face of HIV/AIDS.

The dilemma of the adolescent child was recently captured in a short narration by Tim (not his real name) who said, "Many parents do not know how to deal with the youth. A former classmate of mine was once beaten very seriously by his father when he was found with his girlfriend at their home. The father was away in Nairobi and so my classmate invited his girlfriend over. Unfortunately, the father returned unexpectedly and netted the two. The boy was thoroughly beaten in front of his girlfriend. The young man became frustrated and started taking drugs as a way of rebelling against the father's wishes." Effective media strategies have the ability of helping family members talk with each other. They function as a trigger for family dialogue as well as models on how dialogue within the family could be conducted. This may help Tim's classmate and his parents to understand each other.

Female Circumcision

Female circumcision /genital cut is said to serve a number of functions in communities that undertake it. These include:

(i)   *Rite of Passage:* It marks the transition from girlhood to womanhood. It is symbolic of womanhood because "girls that have undergone it are taught their roles in the community as women and wives. They are taught what to do during pregnancy and childbearing."

(ii) *Restraining female sexuality:* In many cases it is claimed that circumcised women are "sexually disciplined" than their uncircumcised counterparts. It reduces sexual urges and tames the girls.

(iii) *Societal acceptance:* female circumcision in these communities is crucial for girl's acceptability. Circumcised, the girl is viewed as decent and clean; uncircumcised, she is seen as dirty and immoral. She will certainly not expect a man to marry her. Acceptability by community becomes key.

As an attestation of how deep-rooted this practice is, even girls that vehemently condemn it have themselves undergone it, while the boys that also condemn it say they would not get married to uncircumcised girls. Asked why, they respond:

"I would become a laughing stock in my community if I married an uncircumcised girl. I would be seen as a social misfit. All my agemates would not associate with me for they would say that I am married to *etufo* (uncircumcised girl) and not *esiakiki* (a circumcised girl) like them."

And in Kisii, a girl was sent back to her parents from her marital home by her husband so that she could undergo circumcision before she could be accepted as a decent wife. He had discovered that she was not circumcised. When Kisii men are asked whether female circumcision should be banned since it puts girls at the risk of infection because it was carried out in unhygienic circumstances, they say that the girls should be circumcised in hygienic environments using sterilized razors. Makori (not his real name) wonders:

> "Are you really Kisii men? Are you serious about what you are saying or is it because of our visitors? If you are Kisii men and you are genuine with yourselves, you should not cheat the visitors that female circumcision will come to an end in Kisii. While some parents now take their daughters to hospitals, the majority still do it at home. And if you ignore this practice you invite an ancestral curse on your daughters. They may give birth to children who are 'weaklings' or that may die continuously until some cleansing ceremony is done. Is there anyone of you that is prepared to undergo that type of experience and pain?"

From the foregoing, it is clear that there is an urgent need to utilize the mass media, especially the radio, in the efforts to increase levels of knowledge, change attitudes, and influence behavior towards better reproductive health. For maximum results, the drama should target adolescents and young adults especially in the rural areas. Adolescents will listen to programs that are both entertaining and educative. They are resistant to didactic programs. They want information that is packaged in a form familiar and acceptable to them.

Research has shown that even when levels of knowledge are high, there are certain competing trends especially locatable in culture that may hinder the transfer of that knowledge into behavior. Consequently, ways need to be sought in order to address that anomaly through persuasive strategies. In my view, education is not a sufficient condition for behavior change. It needs to be complemented by an appeal to the emotions of the audience. We can do this through serial dramas that are research-based and driven by theoretical understandings of how individuals and communities change.

HIV/AIDS

The HIV/AIDS epidemic is taking a heavy toll on Kenya's economy, development, human resources, and youth. UNAIDS/WHO estimate that over two million adults (15-49) are infected with HIV-- at a rate of nearly 14 percent (UNAIDS/WHO, 2000). Significantly, 62% have heard of people suffering from HIV/AIDS and a similar proportion (67%) know of someone who had died of an AIDS-related illness. The AIDS pandemic has further increased mortality rates, reducing life expectancy by about 12 years for males and over 15 years for females. The gender disparity in infection rates is also evident among the younger population. Studies from Nyanza Province in Western Kenya reveal that 22 percent of young girls between 15 and 19 years of age are HIV-positive, compared with just four percent of their male counterparts (UNAIDS, 1999). The gender disparity in the way HIV/AIDS affects young Kenyans reveals many inequities of cultural, social, and economic factors. Additionally, practices such as early onset of sexual experience, having multiple sexual partners, and low rates of condom use combine to put young people at a higher risk of pregnancy and sexually transmitted infections, including HIV/AIDS. The health and well-being of Kenya's youth are of particular concern not only because of their vulnerability to HIV/AIDS but also because of the central role they should play in the development and future of the country.

The use of entertainment-education approaches to combat HIV/AIDS in Africa is important and urgent. They will have the effect of increasing discussion in communities and working towards informed action. Let me elaborate further.

Entertainment-Education Serial Dramas: The Process

Serial dramas have been used for many years to entertain and educate. When well designed they are a channel through which behavior may be influenced and changed. However, a systematic program design process is necessary. What is this process?

Implementers of this strategy are encouraged to conduct initial research on the critical issues to be addressed. The results are summarized as educational issues which are consequently converted into positive and negative values to be respectively encouraged or discouraged. Main characters who represent positive and negative attributes are designed. In between the two polarities of characterization, are transitional characters who are closest to the target audience in knowledge, attitude and behavior. Characters are rewarded for practising the desired behavior consistently and realistically. Equally, they are punished for engaging in negative behavior. Furthermore, the suggested approach demands that programs be culture sensitive, even as they try to intervene in cultural practices. The key word in all programs is subtlety in dealing with culture.

The drama emanating from the research should be powerful and engaging. Note that drama is about action. The word 'drama' is derived from the Greek word 'dran' which means 'to do'. Drama is a literary composition that tells a story, usually involving human conflict by means of dialogue and action. In other words, drama is supposed to be performed and this can be on stage, television, or radio. Moreover, the performance is always before an audience. It is a re-enaction of situations which have a causal effect on each other with one event or more setting in motion a chain of other events. For instance, the pregnancy of a twelve year old school girl may lead to tensions in the family, separation of her parents, prostitution, sexually transmitted diseases, the establishment of a center for adolescent sexuality and so on.

The difference between a serial drama and regular drama is the duration of the performance. The serial drama is ongoing, open-ended and may be said to be 'never-ending'. An episode opens itself to other future episodes. In addition, in the serial drama, the resolution of conflicts is temporary and leads to the creation of other conflicts. It is like life itself in its continuity, interelatedness and complexity. This continuity is driven by conflict; the center-piece of drama.

The word 'conflict' is derived from the Latin term 'conflictus' which means 'a striking together; a contest'. A conflict is a struggle; a sharp disagreement or opposition, such as of forces, interests or ideas. It is an emotional disturbance resulting from:

♣ a clash of impulses in a person
♣ a clash between people

♣ a clash between an individual and supernatural forces which are uncontrollable.

Dramatic conflict refers to the unexpected and unusual twists and turns which create uncertainty, suspense and tension in an individual or between individuals. The conflict may be due to an uncomfortable sitting together of emotions, events and situations between characters or within a character. For instance, we may experience a conflict if we are equally attracted to two situations and we are obliged to choose one of them. A rural mother who wants to send her daughter to school but is worried that she may lose her to a Western life style is in a state of conflict. This is good fodder for the entertainment education strategy.

Used within the context of popular culture the term 'entertain', derived from the Latin word 'intertenere' means to "engage the attention of", with anything that causes the time to pass pleasantly, such as is done in conversations, music, and drama; to please and amuse. An entertaining experience is one which is pleasant to the emotions. On the other hand, to 'educate' is to give knowledge and skill to someone; to train to develop the knowledge, skill, mind, or character of an individual. When the two terms of entertainment and education are compounded they refer to a type of communication which delivers pro-social messages in a pleasureble way. Therefore, in seeking to educate, messages are deliberately and consistently packaged in a style that is interesting and entertaining.

In Kenya we are anchoring the soap opera as an important way of increasing levels of knowledge, changing attitudes, increasing dialogue in families and communities and influencing the behavior of individuals. In its evolution in the 1920s, the soap opera was first used by American manufacturers of detergents and other household items as a strategy to capture customers, especially women. It was designed on the premise that if the audience was sufficiently attracted by the fictional material in the form of radio drama, they would respond positively to accompanying commercial messages. The argument was that listeners would develop a trusting relationship with the designers of the soap opera and would consequently follow 'suggestions' made about the type of detergent or household goods to buy.

Thus a program format was designed in such a way as to appeal to an audience, largely made of women, and encourage them to listen regularly. The earlier soaps drew heavily on fictional narratives, especially the domestic novel whose main focus was house and home, romance, and familial relationships. For example, they portrayed the conflicts that women experience in balancing family demands, domestic commitments and their own emotional and social needs. At the center of these novels (and by extension, the early soap operas) were women. The popularity of the drama was so immense that it superseded the expectations of the advertisers and sponsors.

The growth of commercial advertising coupled with the extension of radio services nationally contributed significantly in enhancing the soap opera genre. Such soaps as Ma Perkins and *One Man's Family* were broadcast in the 1930s and the long running British Corporation soap operas, including *Mrs. Dale's Diary* (1948-1969), *The Archers* (started 1950) and *Coronation Street* have had a loyal audience. In the 1970s, Miguel Sabido of Televisa argued that although commercial telenovelas had certain values which they transmitted to their audience, they were not consistent. Consequently, there was a need to develop value consistent telenovelas for social benefit. Such telenovelas, Miguel claimed, would encourage pro-social behavior, such as adult literacy and family planning, without being prescriptive. He went ahead to produce telenovelas that were socially beneficial. These included *Ven Conmigo* (Come with Me), *Acompaname* (Accompany Me), *Vamos Juntos* (Let's Go Together), *Caminemos* (Going Together Forward) and so on.

The American Soap *The Guiding Light* began as a radio program in 1937, then in 1952-1956 went out parallel television and radio versions, before continuing in a television only format.

All creative art forms attempt to engage audience members by the posing and working through a complex enigma. The resolution is contained in the text. In soap operas the suspense is deliberately presented, indeed even forced, so that audience members are left waiting for the next episode. The tension that results from the break is captured in the cliff hanger. Audience members are encouraged to ask questions and attempt answers to the complicated plot. In essence, then, the cliff hanger may be crafted as a problem solving process – where audience members are kept in the dark – or audience members can be given limited knowledge on a situation and encouraged to seek further knowledge. Moreover, the serial allows for rare moments of resolution of conflicts and situations.

Characters in soap operas are ordinarily more than one would expect in a stage performance. This creates variety and ensures that they are not "used up" too quickly. They allow wide possibilities for story formulation. However, there is need for a steady and consistent set of characters who push the story forward and with whom audience members can relate, identify and become familiar. But the characters are not the same.

The *individuated* characters have specifically unique traits e.g. overfeeding, cynicism, stinginess, gossip, nagging. Others are character types – negative, positive, transitional – in terms of the values they represent. They share a range of traits recognizable in the large world, outside the soap opera.

There is, of course, the gossip – the character who helps to create the day to dayness of the events in the drama. The gossip makes commentaries on the drama and provides the link between the various story-threads. The gossip within the serial is equally mapped outside it. Audience members gossip about the events in the drama. The soap gives audience members something to talk about as they do other things. Therefore, soap operas provide a strong sense of involvement and this is enjoyable. Further, they stimulate speculative capacities and encourage conjecture.

As never-ending stories, soaps are constantly unfolding narratives, just like life itself. With their slow narrative progression, cliff hangers and tease devices, interwoven storylines and a set of core characters, soap operas can be quite engaging. When imbued with socially relevant and appropriate content, soap operas can contribute to social transformation.

In my view, powerful serial dramas utilize the discourse of persuasion effectively. Persuasion is a verbal method of motivating people's behavior. It plays an important role in effective communication. But how can we do this? I propose the following approaches to writers and producers of health related serial dramas:

(i) Gain and Maintain Attention

A successful soap opera would need to command the attention of it's audience. Generally, attention may be defined as a unified, coordinated attitudinal or muscular set which brings sense organs to bear with maximum effectiveness upon a set of stimulation. Consequently, attention contributes to alertness, and readiness of response in behavioral terms. A socially committed soap opera ought to deliberately work towards commanding the attention of it's audience. How can we command attention?

- *Create Variety:*

Provide variety in setting, character, story, and language. The soap opera format of multiplotlines and different character types provides the writer with variety in character and story. In the act of performance, the producer ensures that the acting varies in mood and presentation.

- *Be Intense*

Both at the levels of writing and acting there should be sustained action. Repetitiveness of situation, action and language lead the audience to a measure of attentiveness which can be reinforced through building layers upon layers of situations and actions. Note that parallelism is a form of repetition and forces us to think about the utterance. It contributes to intensity.

- *Target the Vital:*

Focus on the vital in the lives of your audience. Communicate precisely and unambiguously what is considered important and valuable.

- *Always Contextualize:*

Look around and work through the culture and experiences of your audience. Put everything within context of the speech event. Refer to people, places, objects, and events which are part of the speech situation. This helps create the precise image of the setting in the mind of the audience.

- *Use humor!*

Humor, and its physiological manifestation of laughter, is delightful, entertaining and enjoyable. As a strategy of drawing attention, humor brings gaiety to sombre situations. Humor may be created from funny situations, for instance the stressed out mother may use salt instead of sugar in her tea, or it may stem from the use of double-edged language such as in comedy shows.

(ii) Use strategies of suggestion and subtlety:

Most persuasion uses some type of suggestion, a form of symbol-communication through models, words, pictures or some medium which aims at inducing acceptance of the symbol. In the development of an entertainment education program, a measure of suggestivity is invoked in a number of ways:

- *Prestige suggestion:*

The utilization of celebrities in the serial drama, even if this is only occasional, enhances the prestige of the drama in the eyes of the audience. Detergent and shoe manufacturers use national celebrities to underwrite the merits of their products. Because each soap opera ends with an epilogue the producer can seek the participation of a national celebrity in reading the epilogues as a way of enhancing the image of the program.

- *Ideomotor suggestion:*

Aim at motor reproduction of behavior. It is not enough to introduce ideas into the mind of the listener. The ideas should be supported by a demonstration of how to practise the desired behavior. Motor reproduction is an indispensable component of soap operas for social change. The ideomotor suggestion is a call to action.

- *Indirect suggestion:*

A successful serial drama will desist from overt moralizing. It should, instead, be anchored around subtlety and concealment in the presentation of the values to be enhanced. A classic example of the type of subtlety we have in mind is found in Shakespeare's *Othello*. In that play, Iago cleverly uses Othello's pre-existing inclination towards insecurity and jealousy in order to eventually lead him to accuse his innocent wife, Desdemona, of unfaithfulness. He murders her . The subtle and indirect suggestion is used in order to create an attitude that may lead to future action.

(iii) Develop a favorable atmosphere:
Before the soap opera goes on air, it is important that a favorable atmosphere be created for the program. Among other things, there ought to be favorable publicity and effective introduction of the program. As much as possible, try to have the program aired at prime time for dominance. Peak time differs from country to country. In the course of production, enrich the atmosphere of the program through the use of , among other things, appropriate acoustics and music.

(iv) Establish and maintain common ground:
Right from the beginning of designing the serial, establish a common ground with the audience through analyzing and comprehending their attitudes, beliefs, ideas and interests. This is how to build trust and confidence. Design characters who can bond with your audience because they share a common ground. The audience is, for example, likely to doubt the sincerity of a character who has a superiority complex but is likely to trust a character who speaks their language and idiom and is concerned with their issues. A character who embodies the values to be enhanced in the drama ought to draw the trust and confidence of the audience. Such a character cannot be detached but should be an integral part of the group. Those familiar with the Bible will recall that Jesus Christ became part of the group by using parables to communicate a socio-ethical value.

(v) Cater for the cognitive and affective domains:
Most informational and educational programs target the cognitive domain only. They are interested in transmitting knowledge. But enriching the cognitive domain is not sufficient . In order to persuade the audience to transfer that knowledge to concrete action, it is imperative that programs target both the head (knowledge) and the heart (emotions). This double pronged strategy is more persuasive than the single pronged one.

This critical recommendation for the use of the serial dramas is not without a basis. The experience of the Kenyan serials *Ushikwapo 1 and 2* and *Kuzungumza*, alluded to above, is enlightening and instructive in a number of ways. Both were written in Kiswahili, Kenya's national language, and broadcast at peak time on the national station, the Kenya Broadcasting Service (originally Voice of Kenya). *Ushikwapo 1* was a thirty minute radio soap broadcast twice a week on Mondays and Wednesdays at 12.00 pm, with two subsequent repeats at 6.15pm.

Ushikwapo Shikamana 1 was sponsord by the National Council for Population and Development (NCPD) and was written initially by Kimani Njogu who was later joined the second year of broadcast by the late Kadenge Kazungu. The producer was Tom Kazungu. The program went on air through the Voice of Kenya (currently the Kenya Broadcasting Corporation). It was first transmitted in October 1987 as part of the Information Education and Communication activities of the NCPD.

Ushikwapo 1 highlighted the problems associated with unplanned parenthood (epitomized by Mzee Gogo and his son Kinga), the dangers of promiscuity (exemplified by Shindo and Pambo), the place of inappropriate traditional practices and family harmony. Issues of gender relations within the family were carefully integrated.

According to Alamin Mazrui (1988) after one year of production the program had at least 40% of target audience as regular listeners. Ushikwapo was more likely to produce the desired social change because of its entertainment-education format which allows for experiential learning; and listeners had a more positive attitude towards family planning compared to non-listeners. Ochillo (1990) found out that 61.3% of these interviewed had listened to Ushikwapo 1 and 23% were regular listeners. In Mazrui's findings the percentage of audience members who listened to the program regularly ranged from 22% in Siaya to 50% in Kilifi.

In the Ochillo findings, 40.5% of the regular listeners were between ages 16-25 years and 35.1% were aged 26-34 years. most (47%) had had eight years of education.

This earlier effort at a long range radio soap opera on reproductive health was to give birth to a series of other interventions using a similar format. *Kuelewana* was broadcast once a week for thirty minutes on Sundays at 8.00pm whereas *Ushikwpao 1* was on family harmony, *Kuelewana* was on dialogue within the family. In the late 1980s, there was also a popular television soap on health *Tushauriane* (Let's Advise One Another) which was broadcast once a week. It's discontinuation, due to financial constraints, was the subject of intense parliamentary debate. Around the same time, there was also a television soap opera *Usiniharakishe* (Hurry Me Not) on sexuality behavior. This latter program was discontinued by presidential decree because it was too explicit in its treatment of relationships and was generally viewed as 'culturally insensitive.' Kenya's radio soap operas have had a steady listenership especially in the rural areas where the radio is the main source of information and entertainment, since 1927 when it was first introduced.

It will be noted that the health-related serials I am talking about attempt to be as culturally sensitive as possible and purposefully utilize the language and idiom of the target audience. In these soaps, the events, experiences and idioms are derived from the ordinary people, who also constitute the bulk of the listenership. This is the category that is most vulnerable and urgently requires information that would help them improve their lives in terms of health, education, and economic well-being. Thus, the strategy is to adopt a popular discourse; a discourse that is familiar to the target group.

Just like in real life, characters in health related soap operas are story tellers - stories about themselves and stories about others. Significantly, the production of the Kenyan health related radio serials, with which I have been involved, proceed from the premise that social and cultural problems can be identified and deliberate communication strategies put in place to resolve them. Moreover, it is correctly assumed that the soap opera can be used to change or reinforce the knowledge, attitudes, and practices of listeners. By creating characters who appeal to the world of listeners, serial dramas can influence the behavior of its audience.

The radio drama, as a genre, has a unique style; a style that appeals to the ear rather than the eye and language is used to build the required situation in the mind of the listener. A crucial component of that style is signposting of scene and character. Within dialogue, the sign posting may be achieved through strategic repetition, parallelism, and flashbacks. The dialogue is moreover reinforced by mood music and sound effects in order to create the desired effect in the mind of the listener.

In the case of Africa it is appropriate that the radio be used in the transmission of health messages. The radio, more than the television, is an important tool for the dissemination of health messages in Africa because of its wide reach, affordability and convenience; because it can be used in areas that have no electricity. In dealing with issues of fertility, communication within the family, parental responsibility, gender violence, access to health facilities and treatment of communicable diseases the radio can be key in providing information. Summative research conducted by independent organisations attribute a significant amount of health related behavior change to these soaps. For instance, the radio soap opera -*Ushikwapo Shikamana 1* - listened to by 39 per cent of the country during a midterm survey and upto 61 per cent in a post-transmission survey (Ochillo 1990: 16) increased clinic attendance in rural Kenya. Indeed, the post-transmission survey described the serial as perhaps one of the most effective Information, Education and Communication, program ever to go on air on the Kenya Broadcasting Corporation (Ochillo 1990: 26). A total of 59 per cent found the program to be useful to parents whereas only 2.9 per cent thought the program not useful to parents. This is significant because the main target in the series were young parents. In addition, data from the study indicated that 54.3 per cent of the respondents found the program to be useful to adolescent girls and 50.4 per cent of the respondents found the soap opera to be useful to adolescent boys (Ochillo 1990: 44-45).

The messages communicated in the *Ushikwapo 1* soap opera emphasized monogamy, delaying age of marriage and first childbearing, limiting family size for better health, equal treatment of male and female children, the dangers of promiscuity and unprotected sex, and health problems associated with rapid population growth. Economic issues such as rural-urban migration, unemployment, and the limited agricultural land were also discussed. I would like to argue that beyond the entertainment and educational value of the serials, the drama was acceptable because it utilized the language, idiom and medium of ordinary people.

According to data from a report by Research International, the radio serial *Kuelewana ni Kuzungumza* which was part of the *Haki Yako* (It's Your Right) campaign conducted by the Family Planning Association of Kenya, the serial was heard by approximately 56 per cent of the adult population. Statistics from eighteen family planning clinics showed that new users seen each month increased by 33 per cent - from 1,500 to 2,000 new users. A year after the broadcast began, 76 per cent of the new clients in the eighteen clinics reported listening to the drama, and 38 percent of new clients said the broadcasts influenced them to visit the clinics. By the end of the two-years of the drama, 42 per cent of respondents reported speaking to their spouses or partners about family planning within the last six months. 94 percent of the respondents in the survey stated that it is important to discuss family planning with one's spouse. It will be appreciated that although the approach was appropriately multimedia, the contribution of the radio soap opera was impressive.

A key distinguishing feature of soap story-telling is the organisation of time. The soap tells a complete story but spreads it over a predetermined number of episodes using the cliffhanger device to pick up from one episode to another. The set of unresolved narrative puzzles are used to carry the audience across the time gap. However, the length of the fictional time which is supposed to have passed between episodes is driven by the narrative. Time for the soap is endless but organized. In order to maintain the soap's following, there is every effort to maintain the same time slot for the program.

In soap operas there is a conscious postponement of the final resolutions; unlike the series which has a predetermined number of episodes. It is ongoing and endless life experiences as it opens up all sorts of possibilities: pregnancies open up possibilities of marriage, divorce, marital tensions with the coming of children, marital infidelity, disease and so on. The uncertainty of the future creates suspense and the desire to know; a desire that is increased through the use of the soap opera's traditional hallmark - the cliffhanger. The unfolding of the action in the drama is cut off at a crucial moment so that the riddle is unresolved. One of the reasons for the relative failure of educational programs on matters that have to do with the emotions (such as sexual behavior), is their disregard for the emotional domain in their transmission. In those programs, it would appear that the urge is the transmission of information. I believe that one of the ways of tackling issues that are close to the emotions is to look for a language that speaks to the emotions instead of stating bare facts. Moreover, the message ought to be transmitted in a voice quality that serves as an index of such passing emotional states as happiness, sensuality, optimism.

In the Kenyan radio soaps being used in the promotion of health, there is every effort to be realistic in the portrayal of life, character, and events. However, like all popular culture there is always an element of the melodramatic as a strategy to keep the audience hooked. The trick therefore, is to balance reality with entertainment especially because bare reality is at times not interesting. The stories are structured around a set of issues drawn from research and a values grid which has positive and negative attributes. These values constitute intertextual elements in the drama text. They are statements of truth about life; about experiences.

The discoursal strategy of overtly inserting texts drawn from other sources, sometimes texts from organisations working on health locally and internationally, is what I call, following Fairclough (1992) "manifest intertextuality" and it is intensely used in health related dramas because they are based on a set of issues to be articulated. Characters in this type of drama represent values embedded in two extreme positionalities: there are those who practice the desired behavior and those who fight against it. In between, the two extreme positions characters who are ambivalent, neutral and transitional are developed. In a sense then, like all melodrama, soap drama revolves around the tension between the good and the evil in society.

The soap's longevity and ability to target emotions is useful. It has the ability to create strong identification between audience members and the characters in the drama. It will be appreciated that one of the soap's most striking qualities is the capacity of the audience to become extremely familiar with the history of the main characters and the interrelationships that govern their lives. In a significant number of cases, they are able to pick out the good, the bad and the ambivalent and the values that each character represents in the drama. Identification, as a psycho-social condition of solidarity is vital in behavior change and every effort is made to intensify it in the unfolding of the drama.

One of the important influences of how the audience perceive the soap opera is its regular appearance; in the same slot, every week of the year. The soap attempts to blur the difference between fictional time and real time in the interweaving of storylines. The world of the drama and that of the audience becomes one of neighbors who share experiences, hopes, fears and aspirations. The characters in a serial at the close of an episode pursue an 'unrecorded existence' which may be worked into future episodes or ignored all together. This capacity for the soap opera to temporarily obliterate the distinction between real time and fiction time is truly revealing. It is a facility that the creative team in Kenya uses to move the narrative forward and also to create a sense of reality and identification among the audience. At times the world of fiction and that of reality are collapsed both for practical and theoretical reasons. National events are a times worked into the drama.

Drama is made of events, happenings, and incidents and requires the eye and/or ear of the audience to experience and perceive elements of conflicts and to respond emotionally to these elements of conflict. But to respond emotionally is insufficient for socially committed drama; that type of drama needs to lead to concrete action, to a certain type of behavior and practice. Therefore, for the soap opera to be truly effective as a tool for the promotion of health, it ought to be constructed in a way that the audience can eventually feel close to, identify with, and trust the judgments of the positive models in the drama. It is after a strong bond has been created that health messages are transmitted through the experiences of characters. As the characters in the drama go through a variety of experiences, the audience similarly undergoes the same experiences vicariously. Furthermore, as the characters seek guidance from health centers because of their ailments, so does the audience get motivated to visit the clinic.

It is this unity between sustained behavior in the drama and the real world that gives the desired results. Unfortunately, there is always a general impatience among health workers with the slow unfolding of the drama. They would like to see health messages being transmitted immediately the soap opera starts broadcasting. Whereas this anxiety is understandable, it tends to undermine the theoretical thrust of the soap opera for health promotion. Health messages are best inserted after a bond has been created between the models and the audience, and that takes quite a number of episodes.

Health messages, embedded in the behavior of characters, are subtly communicated through events and experiences. Moreover, some cognitive information is transmitted in the epilogues that come at the end of each episode. Epilogues may be used to answer listeners' questions not on the drama *per se* but on health information regarding where to write or call for assistance. In other words, epilogues are used to transmit cognitive information and they are best delivered by an opinion leader or an individual who represents the best in terms of values and achievement in society. The epilogue makes rational sense of what has transpired in the program, ties the program with the social message, and provides specific information about the relevant social infrastructure.

An important component of health promotion soap operas are letters from listeners. At the end of each episode, listeners are encouraged to write to the program if they have any questions. Normally, in these soaps the questions raised by the audience are either incorporated in the drama or answered by mail. This is an important way of involving audience members in the drama and engaging in dialogue with them.

Conclusion

Thus far, we have seen that the continent of Africa has a number of pressing problems. But these problems can be solved by involving communities. Through entertainment-education communities are given the opportunity to think through these issues. There is therefore a need to continue supporting the different expressions of popular culture so that they can better communicate health messages. In Africa, issues of health are intimately related to poverty and gender. It is imperative, therefore, that pro-health initiatives address questions of poverty alleviation and the status of women. In my view as long as the bulk of the African people continue to live below the poverty line, they will be dogged by diseases, including HIV/AIDS. Moreover, it requires the collaborative efforts of governments, the private sector, and Non-Governmental Organizations to work towards the eradication of gender inequalities and to enhance the status of women in societies, as prerequisites for economic and social development. By providing alternative models and behavior patterns derived from ordinary people and in their own language and idiom, the soap opera has the capacity to sensitize and motivate people towards the creation of a more healthy world. In Kenya such an effort is being anchored around Kiswahili, the national language.

II

It is likely to view the use of forms emanating from the West as a negation of the creative project in Africa. However, this view may be limiting because it assumes that genres are not subjected to cultural interventions once they cross the borders of their origin. Genres are always re-invented and re-crafted. They are never static or insulated.

The soap opera genre has its roots in orature – a phenomenon that exists in all world cultures. With the coming of the genre in Africa, creative writers have continuously extended its limits and redefined its possibilities. Unlike the Hollywood soaps which celebrate excess, individualism and artificiality, the soaps from Africa draw on community values and orature, especially as experienced in performance.

It is this performativity and social consciousness that Micere Mugo exemplifies in her Soap Summit presentation on creativity in Africa.

"Transcending Colonial and Neo-Colonial Pathological Hangovers to Unleash Creativity."

Micere Mugo – Syracuse University

"Thank you very much indeed Dr Njogu for that kind introduction. Allow me to also thank Dr. Onsongo for a very focused speech, especially in terms of the work that is before us at this summit and the president of PCI for the illustrative remarks following the speech.

Let me begin by really expressing deep appreciation for the invitation to come to this soap summit as the keynote speaker. When Dr Njogu invited me, I explained that recently I have been cutting down on my speaking engagements for all kinds of reasons - including health concerns. However, in the end there was no way I was going to say no to Dr. Njogu as he twisted my hand so hard that I ended up accepting to come. Frankly, were it not for health problems, I would never have needed any arm-twisting to accept an invitation to come to Kenya. Just a mention of the motherland would have definitely done the trick!

So, I am really delighted to be with you all and wish to express gratitude to the PCI for funding my travel here. In particular, I want to thank Lillian Chege for shouldering a lot of work in preparing my itinerary, which was a

Culture, Entertainment and Health Promotion

little problematic. Once more, it is truly a pleasure to be at this summit and to have the opportunity of networking with all of you.

Permit me now to become a bit personal and recognize in our midst here two very special people - my sisters. Mrs. Kiereini is a former Chief Nursing Officer in Kenya, currently serving as the Chairperson of AMREF the Board of Directors and Mrs. Marekia is former secretary/office administrator, who is now a businesswoman. Please join me in welcoming them to this soap summit even though they only came to offer me sisterly solidarity by listening to my address. As for all the many friends that I see here and whom I cannot name individually, I embrace each one of you and just want to say how delighted I am to see you at this forum.

At this juncture, I would like to comment in quite some detail on the symbolism of this moment when we find ourselves meeting in Kenya. I feel the need to do so for several reasons that will unfold. But, do not worry! Even though I was given up to one hour to make my remarks, I am going to do my best to cut down on my text because there are some people here who need to get away soon. In fact, I am going to speak to my speech rather than read it out and so if it is a little incoherent please understand that it is because I am trying to be sensitive about taking too much space when time is proving to be such an elusive commodity. Moreover, jet lag has been playing tricks on me and I haven't been sleeping well at all since my arrival. As a result, I am feeling a bit lightheaded.

But, let me move onto symbolism.

The first level of symbolism that I wish to comment on is the tenacity that has made this summit convene at all. Personally, I am quite amazed that it is taking place. Only a week ago, there were e-mail alerts that all international conferences scheduled to take place in Kenya had been canceled for security reasons. Dr. Njogu must have been very vigilant because before I could get onto my computer keyboard to ask him whether the information under circulation was correct, he had sent out an e-mail to all summit participants simply announcing: "the conference is on." That was how brief and decisive his message was. For me, the symbolism here is not to be missed: we have to design our own agenda and move on with it as opposed to taking our queue from others.

You see, the government of George Bush seems to be determining national and personal agenda through security coding – red, orange, yellow and green. There is so much drama around this that it is creating more fear than a feeling of safety. Now, according to this security system, Kenya is a security liability – in fact, a country that poses a serious terrorist threat. So, I am rather surprised to see that many of you are still living here and remain alive. I am happy too to have been here for three days and to be still alive.

Seriously, going by the gravity of these alerts, those of you who live here should presumably have packed your bags by now and fled, while the rest of us would never have boarded the planes to come. But we decided to be crazy and come and it seems that there was some sanity in our madness because we would have been foolish not to come. The lesson is that remaining focused on our agenda and commitments is critical in accomplishing the work that we have mapped out for ourselves.

The second level of symbolism, especially with all these security concerns before us, is that instead of panicking, we should be fired by a sense of urgency to complete the work before us. Speed is critical. It is, in fact, a matter of life and death, particularly when it comes to tackling the HIV/AIDS pandemic, which is more of a source of terror/horror on a day to day basis, more devastating than any terrorist attack we could imagine. Please don't get me wrong, terrorist attacks are lethal and we have already witnessed the extent of their unimaginable terror; but thankfully, in most situations they do not happen every minute of the day. Deaths from HIV/AIDS do. The symbolism of the urgency confronting us becomes a teaching moment, compelling us as artists, culturalists, journalists, writers, activists, etc. We must move forward with all human speed possible. We have to seize every possible moment to intervene in order to avert this human calamity that has gone out of control.

The third level of symbolism – that of the larger historical Kenyan scene – calls for a special, prolonged comment. Please allow me to indulge. I am entering this country for the first time since the December elections that toppled the Moi dictatorship and for once, I am encountering people with a lot of hope. I am thrilled by it, but I am also reminding all of us to remain cautious and vigilant. This is because as we know, we have lived through euphoria before only to experience huge let downs. However, we do not want to feed on pessimism: we want to say that things will go right - that we will make them go right. Yes, for the first time after so many years, I am seeing and hearing people express confidence in their ability to create positive change. So, I want to suggest that symbolically, we meet in Kenya at the dawn of a new day and depending on what action we take, we can make a difference that will affect tomorrow. We have met here to propel change and to make a difference. Let us not forget, however, that to be of lasting transformation, the change we make must be collective. This is the symbolism that we can draw from Kenya where we are meeting under a new political dispensation created through the collective will of the people. If we forget the collective nature of this victory and its significance, we will have betrayed history all over again. This will be yet another political disaster.

We have met here to find ways of working together collectively in order to address the countless problems facing us in Africa. As we look at these problems, we sometimes become discouraged and do not know where to begin; yet we know that we need to begin somewhere. I don't know if all of you suffer from this momentary panic, but I do.

The fourth level of symbolism for me is the celebration of people's potential in changing the oppressive reality facing them. In Kenya and other countries where windows of democracy have opened up, people have every right to bask in the sunshine ushered in by a new dawn, emerging as it does after a long night of terror. We have the right to enter the spaces we have created in order to enjoy the sunshine that we have been a part of the making and to affirm the fact that the sun's rays will stretch into the future. So, overwhelming as the task is, let us take comfort in the fact that daylight is on our side!

Having highlighted these levels of symbolism, let me now celebrate all those who have come to this soap summit as creators of one kind or another: artists, who use their imagination to fathom and create new worlds while believing in infinite possibilities; journalists, who have been so vigilant in naming the ills of neo-colonialism; activists, who have been the voice of our collective conscience especially under silencing; others from various professions who have given their skills to make a difference...Yes, I want to celebrate all of you who are here in the name of naming ourselves and our reality, and in the spirit of making things happen as we all struggle to introduce sanity in a world gone mad. I salute you, fellow travelers, who have chosen to use action to fight pessimism, for we have witnessed the shedding of too many tears.

I truly celebrate the wealth of imagination represented here and just want to give an inspirational speech to say I believe we can change the oppressive reality before us as well as our people. Yes, we can do it. We must believe that as human beings, we have the capacity to transform our world. In celebrating you as cultural agents, I also celebrate our art and cultural heritages. I say, we have here a harvest of multifarious talents and we saw clear evidence of this earlier on in the morning during the opening session. It really was delightful and instructive listening to the members of the opening panel who covered so many issues with such stunning creativity that they have made my task a lot easier. All I need to do now is fire your enthusiasm rather than advice you on what to do. In fact, I am going to narrow my remarks to address the theme of "Transcending Pathology Created by Colonialism and Neo-colonialism in Order to Unleash Creativity." My argument is simple, until we recover from colonial and neo-colonial pathological hangovers, we cannot create meaningful soaps to address other health issues. Hopefully, the challenges I pose will provide a framework around which to brainstorm on how to move beyond borrowed solutions in order to emerge with our own inventions.

Let me now invite you to participate in the rest of my delivery, as I happen to be a child of **orature** and so believe in audience participation. In orature style, when I speak I don't take the audience for granted. I like having them accompany me on our joint conversational journey. So I am going to give you a cue, indicating where you are supposed to come in. The one I am going to use employs a South African term, "abantu," which simply means "people." When I call upon you: "Abantu!" You are going to respond, "ii!" (Gikuyu term for "yes") telling me you are there. Then I will ask you," Shall I go on?" "Shall I proceed?" Shall I speak?"...and/or other such variations. You will respond: "ii!" or "Yes!" However, if you say "No!" I will stop. So, any minute really that you feel tired, you know what to do. But please don't stop me too soon: let me speak for a few minutes at least.

"Abantu!"

"ii!"

"Shall I begin?"

"ii"

I want to begin by stressing that as we celebrate life and the possibilities before us, we are also situated amidst poverty, disease and other calamities. We convene here at a moment when there are so many wars – actual and metaphorical – raging in Africa. A lot of our children are dying, while others have been turned into child soldiers in unending ugly wars of hatred, bloodthirsty power mongering and wanton destruction of lives. In the words of Ambassador Olara Otunnu, the Undersecretary General of the United Nations, our children are being taught to kill while being killed before they have time to grow. This is a tragedy, especially when we think of the AIDS epidemic and other killer diseases such as malaria, cancer and so on that are wiping out our people. So, this is a critical moment for us as artists, culturalists and activists to ask: how can we address these issues? How can we use our imagination to bring creativity to these spaces where there is death and destruction?

"Abantu!"

"ii!"

"Am I making sense?"

"ii!"

"I was nervous that someone would say "no" there because I am not really sure I am making sense."

With these serious challenges in view, I suggest that we do all in our power to move beyond symptoms and get to the root of the problems identified. Above all, we need to have a clear understanding of "where the rain began to beat us," to borrow the words of Chinua Achebe. I repeat: it is critical that we understand where, when and why our problems started. Important as this question is, it seems that when some of us raise it there are people who become nervous, asking, "Why do we have to dig up these past issues? Why don't we just forget?" This self-imposed amnesia is another very severe illness that we have suffered from since colonial times. We are afraid to recall what went wrong, partly because the act of remembering forces us to step in and take action to remedy the offending situation. I want us to remember. I want to take you through some painful moments, not for sadistic reasons, but because they will jerk our memories to remember why we are having so many things going wrong scores of years following independence. How can Africa, a continent that had so much hope at independence reek out so much helplessness? I remember the optimism we had when we came out of Makerere in the 1960s. We were so very full of hope. We were so sure we would make things happen. We were full of commitment. We were going to serve the continent as teachers, doctors, nurses, lawyers, architects, engineers, writers and so on. We must ask: "Where did the rain begin to beat us? What went wrong?"

For sure a lot of blame goes to our leaders, especially those who have ended up becoming dictators, for, at their hands we have witnessed untold terror and destruction, especially that of human resources. However, as ruthless and pathetic as African leaders have been, the people of Africa must assume collective responsibility for having been largely silent while these destroyers ravaged our countries and resources. Yes, it is a shame that at first only a few people dared to speak out against these crimes. If the entire continent had spoken out loud, do you think these dictators would have had enough jails in which to lock all of us up? That would not have been possible and probably change would have come a lot sooner. Look at the collective psychological trauma this inaction has resulted in! Our countries need therapy. It is indeed my sincere hope that the soaps we create will address these issues of psychological health. Our collective humanity has been brutalized by what has happened over time. The soaps will have the challenge of indicating ways of giving birth to new human beings with a vision and mission that seeks to humanize the entire world.

Having said that, I want to believe that there is a reason we have gone through so much pain and that hopefully, we have learnt a lot through our mistakes. In this regard, I must celebrate the people of Kenya and others from all over Africa for deciding to rise up in the end and say, "No! We are not going to allow terror to continue. We are bringing humiliation to a stop in order to move forward!"

"Abantu!"
"ii!"
"Shall I proceed?"
"ii!"

As we try to understand what went wrong, let us not underestimate the impact of an internalized colonial ethos and how the psyche it created shaped the people that we find in ourselves today. But then, some of you will say to me that this is placing blame on colonial masters, turning them into convenient scapegoats. But let me tell you: to understand ourselves fully, we have to comprehend our past. If we don't understand colonialism and the way it worked in order to leave us in the neo-colonial mess that we find ourselves in, we are failing to understand a very important part of our history. Yet, only proper understanding will help us move forward meaningfully into the future.

We are talking of behavior change at this summit. In my view, there is no way I can deal with this question without revisiting colonialism. For, if former colonial subjects are to employ behavior change theory to their lives, they must have the courage to go back to colonization and analyze the consequences of a colonial mentality victimology.

This is the only way we can transform the legacy of abuse, self-doubt (even self-hatred), and an incurable pre-occupation with Whiteness as a coveted state of being. Ladies and gentlemen, those of you coming from a colonial background may not want to hear this, but I want to suggest that we are still suffering from a colonial hangover that has been re-enforced under neo-colonialism. We have grown to not only lose confidence in ourselves, but in our history and culture. Thus, as we seek to create change through soap operas, we need to revisit these abandoned sites - not in a spirit of nostalgia - but in active search of culturally homegrown solutions to our specific, local problems. We need to love ourselves, understand ourselves and re-embrace our heritage. Why? Because when a person really understands himself or herself, when a person has the language and words to name herself/himself and her/his world, then s/he is in control. But once you don't have a language; once you don't have a past; when you pass a vote of no confidence in yourself, you lose the ground on which to stand in order to be sufficiently grounded to transform your reality as necessary.

Let me give an illustration. In the last three days that I have been here, I have been looking at television and 90% of the time the programs that are on the screen are from the west - Europe, Britain, or North America. I am asking myself, "How is this so on a continent where creativity is in so much abundance that we should not be knowing what to do with it? How do our people see themselves in the faces that are on these screens? How do the exhibited Hollywood scenes and the reality show characters of the Gerry Springer drama, for instance, reflect Africa's crying needs? What is going on? For me, there is an obvious problem here, especially for children who are always on the look out for models. It is as if we are telling our children that they ought to look outside themselves, their societies and their worlds in their struggle to construct their identity.

People, there is a crisis here - a big crisis - and I am calling upon all of us to speed up the production of locally generated and oriented soaps in order to speak to Africa's needs. Where urgency is concerned, I am in agreement with the donors. We need to make those soaps happen today: we needed to have done so yesterday. On the other hand, however and this is critical, the work must not be done at the cost of cultural authenticity. We must be careful, even as we rush production, to ascertain that whatever is done is rooted in and mirrors the cultural understanding and self-reflection of our people. I am agreeing that there's urgency and the struggle is at a phase when we really need to speed up action, but not at a cost to our integrity.

"*Abantu!*"

"*ii!*"

"*Shall I proceed?*"

"*ii!*"

With your permission, I will revamp my theorization further and take you back to the question of the urgency in rooting out colonial mentality. I insist that to address Africa's ills we have to begin with attacking the psychological block that undermines our self-confidence, making us always want to look for answers from the outside. Until we learn to trust the strength, the imagination, the will and the creativity within ourselves – to have abundant faith that we can make things happen, we will continue to helplessly gaze outwards. You see as agents of change, we have to be creative, we have to move from the colonial mentality of self mutilation, self destruction and self doubt – erase from our psyche the culture of self-contempt and even self-hatred, a malady that makes us imagine that whatever we have is inadequate and inferior to things western. We have to work towards the rehabilitation of our mutilated, dismembered personal and collective self-imaging and come to trust that we have within ourselves the human potential for determining our lives. The inculcation of an inferiority complex among the colonized was a clear goal in colonial education. It happened in India, it happened here, it happened everywhere colonials set foot and it continues to take place under neo-colonialism. We cannot afford to delay the process of creating soaps that will undo this psychological damage/mischief even as we campaign against other visible medical illnesses and health concerns.

There's a very revealing documentary entitled, *In the white man's image* that narrates the tragic story of North American Indians and the way they were colonized through the elimination of their identity as well as culture. In the documentary there is a ruthless White educator who makes it his mission to not just educate Indian children but to actually change them, mentally and physically. There is a very chilling recurring line in which the colonizer constantly speaks of the need to "kill the Indian and save the man" – obviously meaning there is a need to erase the Indian in the children by turning them into Whites. This process of "killing" the Indian is equivalent to exorcising the "native" out of colonized Africans. Within this context, the victims had to be given new names when they entered government or missionary schools under colonialism. In my case I ceased to be Njiru or Micere and became "Madeleine," acquiring a French name that I could not even pronounce then! So, at one point in my primary school life I was known as "Madeleine Richards." This would be my name at school and on returning home I would revert to my African name – pick up my identity. In this bizarre situation, some people ended up having double personalities and developed a rather schizophrenic relationship with themselves, their homes, their culture and their identity. Serious stuff!

All of this partly explains why an identity crisis persists among our youth, including those who have never left their homes - yet experience a deep craving for wanting to be either American, or British, or anything that is not African. We have passed on the confusion to them under neo-colonialism. It always surprises me when I hear the older generation accusing the youth of losing their culture and identity. Rather than blame them, we should be laying the responsibility on the collective social ethos of self-devaluation that has emerged over historical times. I say, when we begin with a lack of self-knowledge, we are not in a position to become agents of change. The situation is not getting any better, much as we may pretend it is. As we speak, there is a project of re-colonization afoot, which comes as a part of the globalization package. We need to be fully aware of what the process is all about in real practical terms. Namely, that there is now a single power – America – supported by the international corporate world and dominating the rest of the globe, with poor nations at the bottom of the rubble. Let us not mince words: President Bush of America is out to conquer the rest of the world and to colonize weak states. I am cautioning that this culture of dominating others militarily, economically, politically and culturally is the philosophy behind globalization. We need to be keenly conscious of this.

Some people have been as bold as to openly advocate the re-colonization of Africa. There was a very revealing article in the *New York Times* around the mid 1990s in which a scholar by the name of Johnson was proposing that Africa was better off under its former masters and that it was high time ex-colonial powers returned to re-colonize the African continent. Now, nobody is disputing the fact that neo-colonial African leaders have turned the continent into a basket case. There is indeed a sense in which the dictatorships we have survived - not to mention the general mismanagement of our resources - have dragged Africa many years back. In Kirinyaga, for instance, where I come from, roads that were in excellent functioning order during the 1960s and 1970s are no longer passable. There was a road between Kutus and Kibirigwi on which I used to drive at about 40-50 m.p.h. in my little Volks Wagon beetle traveling from Kabare High School to Nyeri, but now that road cannot even carry a donkey cart. This state of things is unacceptable. Yet, in the midst of all this, some African rulers have been known to boast of how much they own. You no doubt know the story of the late Mobutu sese seko who became furious and insulted when a journalist asked him if it was true that he was the tenth (or some such rank) richest man in the world while he was actually much richer than that. Mobutu nearly swallowed the poor journalist alive! Oh the nerve! Some thief is here, having impoverished his country and having grabbed everything that there is to grab and he is boasting about being a better thief than estimated! Friends, I am saying that there's a lot of work to be done because to a certain extent we have called upon ourselves the contempt with which we are being treated. But, even with all of this granted, who is Mr. Johnson to decide to choose the future for Africa! How does what has happened under neo-colonialism make colonialism right given all the dehumanization and suffering it unleashed on African people?

The above reminds us that soap operas have a role to play in filling in the gaps that exist and in exposing the ills that Africa ails from today. If we do not do this, someone else will step in and fill the gap. In cultural terms, this is already happening. At the levels of television, film and media alone, for instance, re-colonization is a real threat.

Let me give you an example. Go to any part of the world be it in Africa, Latin America, Japan, the Caribbean, etc., and you will find that one of the clearest television stations is CNN. The whole world is being brought up on CNN. Now, I have nothing against CNN, nor cross-cultural convergence of resources for that matter. In fact I was watching CNN only this morning when I lost sleep! What I am saying is that when you go to a country and cannot access programs on the local station because CNN has the clearest beam, then there is a problem. What we are witnessing is the equation of globalization with mainstream 'Americanization' and this, in essence, constitutes global colonization. I am arguing that there is something dangerously wrong when the world falls under the superpowership of one country. We need independent film and media to provide an alternative, especially for Africa's and the world's poor. This new imaging created by independent media must strive to gather together all cultures and all people – irrespective of race, class and gender – making them a part of global humanity.

There's a problem here and it is among the root causes that we are needing to address in our artistic products if we are going to make headway.

"Abantu!"

"ii!"

"Are you tired?"

"No!"

"Don't say yes, just yet. I promise I am coming to an end!"

So, what is the way forward? As we struggle to wean ourselves of the colonial and neo-colonial hangovers that I have talked about, we must simultaneously work on creating alternatives. Soap operas have a very special role to play in this task, as already intimated. Only such alternatives will bring about an alternative form of development – one that focuses on entire human populations rather than on a few privileged individuals. We must move beyond self and realize that without collective development, no given country can make the mark. In the prophetic words of J.M Kariuki - a popular politician assassinated in the 1970s (speaking in reference to Kenya): "We do not want a [country] with ten millionaires and twenty million beggars." Those of us who are socially privileged ought to seriously take heed of these words. Africa today has armies of poor people while a small elite wallows in obnoxious wealth. This will take us nowhere. Sometimes you wonder how most people live from day to day- how they survive.

Last night I went to bed very humbled and deeply pensive. I had sat next to a young man at dinner (I hope he is here), who told me his story of survival and human triumph. He was born in Mathare Valley, where he grew up - largely in the streets - living on an empty stomach most days. I don't know how he survived, but today he is here as one of our participating artists and community activists. I was simply amazed by his story and even more so, by the determination with which emerged out of a human pit where so many others of our children have gone down.

I am trying to say that there is something grossly wrong when we have armies of children in the streets; when so many are homeless and hungry; when sprawling ghettos become eye sores and yet we remain surrounded by so much wealth. There's clearly something wrong when we are plagued by so much illiteracy - having to deal with people who cannot decipher an iota on paper - while there are so many of us who are educated. It is in view of all this that I am persuaded there is no other way outside collective development. I am positing that for those of us who are privileged, our privilege is also a responsibility. On this score, Mwalimu Njogu, I celebrate you for having organized this gathering to remind us that we owe the world a responsibility by putting us to work on doing something concrete to change the status quo.

"I am because you are and since you are, therefore I am." This is a rough quotation from John Mbiti's *African Philosophy and Religion* and teaching that we find in most African orature heritages. I subscribe to it – heavily! I tell you, don't you listen to anyone who suggests to you that this kind of thinking belongs to "primitive" and/or "communist" societies. Every human being should have this as a life motto.

Allow me to belabor the point and ask that we remember we did not make it to where we are alone; that in actual fact we are products and extensions of our communities and that, above all, we are products of the years of historical struggles waged by people before us. Sacrifices liberated a lot of the spaces that we occupy to day. The soaps we create must, therefore, address the dangers of individualistic development. Our soaps must never get tired of naming the dangers of poverty and disease. Indeed, they must make a connection between poverty and insecurity; between impoverishment and disease, etc. They must ask harsh questions regarding the role of the World Bank, IMF and imperialist domination – all of which create an indebtedness that makes the poor of the world even poorer. Above all, acknowledging the importance of collective development, please I beg us all to leave behind existing divisions based on all petty nonsense related to tribalism, ethnicity and other socially created barriers such as gender inequity and discrimination against those with disability, etc. We must never ever forget the tragedy of the Rwanda genocide, of Burundi, the DRC, Sierra Leone, Kenya's Rift valley massacres and so on. While on this point, let me say that I can never understand how/why - with all our problems in Africa, including the scourge of killer diseases - we succumb to the madness of sharpening machetes, pangas, arrows, spears and loading guns for killing other people simply because some lunatic of a power hungry warlord convinced us they should die since they don't come from the same group as us!

Sometimes I have wondered, what happened to our psyche? Why have African lives been rendered so cheap...so easily dispensable? Look at this morning's newspaper and see what happened in Mathare Valley yesterday! Why would a landlord exploit unemployed youth to go and evict tenants by beating them, just to get them and others killed in the process? Where is this kind of individualized greed and thuggery going to take us? These are all serious questions that our soaps must pose. To quote Chinua Achebe, "the house is on fire!" I am referring to the analogy he gave in one of his essays regarding a man whose house was ablaze and as it was burning down, he saw a rat running away to escape the fire. And you know what the stupid man did? Instead of focusing on rescuing his belongings, he took a huge stick and began chasing after the escaping rat. I recount this story and have done so several times before to suggest, ladies and gentlemen, that Africa - our "house" - is on fire. Please do not let us go chasing rats that are intelligent enough to escape the fire. There are far too many 'rats' that we keep chasing even as our house burns: petty "tribalism," ethnicity; political war games; idle consumerism; competitive parading of wealth exhibits and so on.

In this regard, let us vow to make the soaps we create focus on the core issues that affect the lives and health of our Africa's majorities most. In creating the soaps, we should engage the question of local languages and involve the masses in the creation of the pieces. Let the people speak for themselves by telling their own stories wherever possible. We cannot possibly replace their voices, however talented or skilful we may be artistically. I keep emphasizing that until we network with the masses in the production of knowledge and other cultural products, intellectual output is going to remain the monopoly of the elites. In this respect, we should recognize the criticality of Orature. In African orature we have an incredibly rich heritage that we should truly be proud of. It has an abundant reservoir of stories; allegories; epics; songs, etc. that will greatly enhance our creativity. I remember how at the height of political repression here in Kenya, one of the dramatists (I forget what his name was) used animal characters types to populate his political satires. These characters represented real people on the Kenyan political scene – roaming the stage as hyenas, elephants, ogres and so on. Once, a senior government minister that I will not name lavishly praised this use of African culture, little knowing that he was one of the undesirable animal characters on the stage that day. We sniggered all the way from the National Theater to the Norfolk hotel where we enjoyed tea and jokes at his expense! Orature is a goldmine and a powerful artistic tool at our disposal whether we are operating from the rural areas or urban set ups. This was ably illustrated during the opening panel to day.

The application of orature in creating soaps and other artistic products will serve a useful purpose in bringing out the interdependence between ethical and aesthetical concerns and this foregrounds the old time debate regarding "art for art's sake" and functional creativity. In orature conceptualization, there is no contradiction, for, it is not a question of either/or, but rather a matter of complementariness. This is to say that in orature, while art is by and large utilitarian, its aesthetic appeal also matters. The orature heritage perceives art as an aspect of human productivity that has a functional purpose, but one that is also meant to express beauty while it entertains the audience. Thus, when we describe soaps as edutainment, we are at one with the orate tradition in which teaching, education and entertainment converge to define a desirable piece of art.

As we compose, script and produce our soap operas, let us not forget to inco-orporate the youth as a target audience. If we are not careful, the marginalization of youth in many of our undertakings is going to cost us heavily somewhere along the way. There is an illustrative story that reinforces the aspect of behavior change theory that posits that habits

Culture, Entertainment and Health Promotion

inculcated early in life are likely to have a more lasting effect on a growing child. The story has it that a Catholic priest was asked by his Anglican counterpart: "How come the Roman Catholic has such a huge, loyal following?" The Catholic priest replied, "Aah! We catch them when they are young!" Please, let us catch them when they are young and if well done, the messages we pass through the soaps we create will rub on, becoming life lessons. Returning to orature yet again, the heritage has genres that naturally attract the attention of young people, especially song and dance. Look at the phenomenal role the two have played all over Africa, especially in liberation struggles!

Only last December, the Kenyan political landscape was a theater using orature popular art forms to mobilize the people. There is a song that I became so addicted to after my nephew played it in the car for hours that I seem to be constantly singing it in America six months later. I am referring to "Yote Yawezekana"…"Everything is Possible"…without you know whom – no need to mention names! The notion of people embracing their self-empowerment and declaring that they are capable of creating any type of change without dictatorial blocks is most refreshing after so many years of silencing. Soaps should exploit the orature genres of dance and song as they naturally appeal to young people and tend to unleash their creativity while enlisting participation without too much of an effort.

In conclusion, let me echo the spirit of this song and say that in the work before us, having shed off colonial and neo-colonial hangovers and then fortified ourselves with self-knowledge and determination, "yote yawezekana!" So, next time you wake up feeling defeated and tempted to remain between those sheets, just throw off the blanket and tell yourself, "I am unbwogable!" (to evoke another popular election song in which the opposition was vouching, "we shall not be moved!") Let us harvest this field of fertile imagination all around us and get on with creating those overdue soaps and other popular art forms that we need for moving our work forward.

Let us remind ourselves time and again: we can do it! We will do it!

"Abantu!"

"ii!"

I will stop now. Thank you very much.

III

History of Entertainment Education in Africa

Although the phrase 'entertainment-education' may be fairly new, the manifestation of this duality of artistic production has long been appreciated. In orature, artistic productions were entertaining and educative. It is within this context that a panel was constituted to reflect on the background to entertainment-education in Africa.

(The panel consisted of Femi Jarret, Executive Producer ARDA Nigeria; Kimani Njogu, Regional Representative, PCI Kenya; Herbert Makoye, Department of Fine and Performing Arts, University of Dar es Salaam, Tanzania. The session was chaired by Oby Obyerodhiambo who wondered whether there has been a time when entertainment in Africa has not been issue based and when was it never useful?)

Femi Jarret, began his presentation on *Background for Soap Opera in Africa* by narrating two folk stories titled *"All of us"* and *"Epelepe Furo"*. He then pointed out that in order to entertain you must have an audience. "Human beings seem to desire pleasure more than they do information. The solution is to make the messages or information a part of the show. Our forefathers in Africa were aware of this, hence our oral traditional art of story. In order to keep the audience captivated, songs, dances, and the whole gamut of theatre have long been used for the dissemination of cultural and social information, values and norms, like the stories he had just narrated. The thrust of these stories was to encourage members of the community cultivate positive moral values.

Storytelling can be used to re-enact the horrible reign of kings and greedy rulers in a way that even the kings would cringe at some of the atrocious things depicted in the play. The storytelling could easily recourse to animal characters to avoid being too obvious and too confrontational.

Ancient communicators like the Greeks, Romans, Hebrews and some of our forefathers in Africa knew that "in order to teach, someone must be listening" (Christine Bailey, 1994). In order to command the attention of the audience, the messages or information should not subsume the story (or entertainment).

In contemporary times, Nigeria has faced the most outrageous political repression carried out by the military dictators. Media freedom and free expression were routinely abused and suppressed. The junta and the media clashed often; because, the media portrayed the grave political situation and highlighted issues of human rights abuses, corruption, state unresponsiveness and lack of accountability. Most press centers and media houses had their offices sealed for disagreeing with the government or for not couching their media messages within the confines of what junta felt was good press. And since government had monopoly of the electronic media ownership, access to radio or TV by opposing voices was denied.

The onerous, yet, seemingly, insurmountable challenge of highlighting the social and political realities in Nigeria without seeming offensive, led to an upsurge in creative initiative to adapt to the inclement political terrain in the country.

The African Radio Drama Association (ARDA), a non profit, non governmental development communication organization for instance, had to rely on entertainment to educate, communicate and promote social change. ARDA, designed and developed radio Soaps geared towards promoting positive change in politics, economic and health issues. Programs were packaged in languages that are easily understood by Nigerians: Rainbow City, a drama in Pidgin English (the "lingua franca" of rural and urban dwellers in Nigeria), "Asuba Ta Gari" meaning "A New Dawn" in Hausa, "Orogojigo" which means "Deep and Wide Matters" in Yoruba and "Chiefoo" meaning "Daybreak" in Igbo language, are examples of the serial ARDA broadcasts daily on over 25 radio stations in the country.

Drama is particularly effective in motivating behavioural change. It not only entertains, but also educates and promotes positive change in behaviour. Stories in form of satire can be used in contemporary Africa to highlight societal maladies without offending the sensibilities of the government. We must remember that although most governments are democratic in their pronouncements, there are still undercurrents of autocracy and intolerance for criticism and opposition. In Nigeria, despite laws permitting private ownership of all media, receiving approval for a license is like getting a camel through the proverbial needle. Few private stations exist, and public radio is seen as the property of the government in power. Thus, getting programs that draw attention to the problems of society caused by leaders will be barred from the stations. This is where drama helps not only to entertain but also to educate."

The second panelist was Kimani Njogu who made a presentation titled *Dancing with information.* He began by pointing out that issue-based entertainment preceded the colonial encounter and was basically captured in orature: the longer narratives and stories, the proverbs, riddles, the performances at social events. He went on: "There was the masquerade in West Africa associated with the construction of social categories and legitimization of authority. There were the griots among the Madinke and Wolof (djely and djely mousso). There were poetic competitions in dialogue form such as Kibati in Pemba and gicandi, among the Gikuyu. These were creative pieces drawn from the cultures. They functioned as commentaries on society. The commentary could also be manifest in the rites of passage, such as on the entry to adulthood and at death, characterized by the carnivalesque, the tentative suspension of social prohibition. Storytelling was an integral part of our lives and it could take quite different forms and used indigenous instruments to accompany the narratives.

With the entry of colonialism, naturally issue based entertainment started utilizing cultural instruments and processes from the West. There were the concert parties: high life West Africa, Taarab in East African coast. The growth of tourism, mining camps and the ghettos also made possible the emergence of a fusion of African cultural productions with the West creating what may be called Afro-European performance culture, such as the South African isicatamiya among the Zulu made contemporary by Lady Smith Black Mambazo.

This fusion between indigenous story telling forms and other forms from the East and West has gained momentum within the postcolonial era and so much with the intensification of globalization. Hybridity and the carnival have become, at least for me, the way to understand African artistic productions.

The youth are dancing through life! Issue-based entertainment is especially appropriate for the youth. African youth are not likely to be influenced by documentaries and research reports. They are not impressed by rigorous analyses, told painfully. Teenage entertainment invariably plays cultural and educative roles that the commercial sector has exploited effectively. In Africa, young people are learning about sexuality and relationships less from established institutions – the family, school, church and more from their peers. They feel they are self sufficient in order to keep adults at bay; but even more importantly, although less appreciated as a result of content and emotions generated from commercial entertainment. They are attracted to romantic love and sexual feeling - falling in love, falling out of love. Entertainment for the youth expresses adolescent emotional dilemma; a dilemma that has elements of realism and fantasy.

Teenage culture - expressed in music, dance, dress, walking and standing habits, facial expression and slang is tending towards the non-verbal and to be image driven. Teenagers are no longer very interested in informational programming - instead they have drifted into the culture of leisure. This is the space, where more programming could take place in order to ensure the consistency of socially positive and culturally sensitive manner. But to be culturally sensitive is not to celebrate all aspects of cultural production. Rather, it is to be conscious of what culture could offer in order to ensure acceptability, longevity and legitimacy.

Globalization and the mushrooming of FM stations have ensured the existence of a vibrant teenage culture. But Africa runs the danger of being swallowed in this wave of uncritical acceptance of everything foreign. Through deliberate development of local interventions, which take into account critical national issues and the emerging teenage culture, we are able to facilitate more relevant and socially functional programming. In my view such programming ought to be guided by cultural sensitivity.

Drawing from my experience and writing with others on over 200 episodes of *Ushikwapo Shikamana* (1986 - 1989) *Kuelewana ni Kuzungumza*

(Nov. 1992 - 1995; 136 episodes); *Ushikwapo Shikamana* (1997 to 2004) and helping in the design of *Twende na Wakati* (1993 to present); *Mambo Bomba* (2003, ongoing) in Tanzania; *Usigo Unnake? Sarivolana* in Madagascar and *Romadi* in Eritrea as well as other soaps globally, I feel that we can use soap operas to influence any social, economic, environmental and political issue. But the effectiveness of our presentations will be dependent on a number of things. These may include:

(a) Cultural sensitivity and appropriateness;
(b) Basing programming on research at various levels;
(c) Constructing effective stories, which go beyond the realistic, and inviting audience to imagine an ideal world for the organization of relationships; powerful stories that have twists and turns at times quite unpredictable.
(d) Creating powerful female characters;
(e) Taking an optimistic posture and giving hope to communities.
(f) Adopting a multimedia strategy that incorporates discussions, cartoons, and listening groups, among other segments.

Our soaps invite the audience to an ideal world; a world different from what they experience everyday. Yet what is it that we want the African audience to imagine? In *Dynasty* we are presented with costumes, décor, and setting chosen for look and feel (not appropriation of plot) luxury, abundance of Western capitalism quite evident despite the sadness; material fulfillment amidst a moral void.

And *Dallas, the Young and Restless, Bold and Beautiful*, like *Dynasty*, pose the challenge: "what would it be like to have all material needs met; to conquer scarcity and enjoy abundance?" It is almost as if the audience believes that by devouring the spectacle, their wants will vanish; consumption, as spectacle, is an approximation of a utopian situation. Is this the type of utopia we want the African audience to imagine?

The dominant feature of the soaps designed in the US and consumed in Africa is more and more abundance and excesses. The British soaps on the other hand, are pegged on community, especially through the rituals, which mark major events in *Coronation Street* and *EastEnders*, for example. As Christine Geraphy (1991) observes:

"It is clear that the ideal community only functions if women are in control: they bring isolated and desperate individuals into the community/family; they organize its rituals; they transmit its values; and spin the web of gossip through which it is continually renewed."

Community is presented as an ideal worth pursuing. That sense of community seems to also inform African soaps such as *Twende na Wakati, Kuelewana* and *Ushikwapo Shikamana*. Soaps are experienced at home either individually or within the family but they do get into the communities through discussions among friends, acquaintances and strangers. They give communities something to talk about. The sharing is not just information; it is also emotional. Soaps can be used to negotiate difficult situations and dilemmas through a blurring of the fictional and the real.

It is clear from these reflections that more social programming will use entertainment in Africa. The biggest challenge that we are likely to have is how to ensure consistency of message; much as we emphasize entertainment. How, for example, do we ensure that popular artists contribute in the enhancement of the status of women by portraying an alternative world other than perpetuating stereotypes? Or how do we ensure that the presentation of fantasy is supported by notions of individual and collective efficacy; a recognition that we can make a difference in our lives; the invocation of a critical and responsible consciousness? These are some of the challenges that issue-based entertainment in Africa will have to contend with."

Herbert Makoye, in his presentation *Tale-Telling Tradition Techniques in Africa and Soap Opera: The Case of Tanzania*, began by saying that the successes and high rate of adoption of radio soap operas in Tanzania and how fast the form has grown in a short time raises a lot of questions, which need to be answered. In his discussion, however, he tried to deal with one question: *why radio soap operas have became so dear to Tanzanians* and the international and local NGOs in a short time of its existence.

He gave a brief history of soaps in Tanzania and pointed out that they started ten years ago (in 1992/1993) when *Twende na Wakati* was created. "This radio soap was created basically to promote family planning and improve family welfare among Tanzanians. The government of Tanzania and United Nations Population Fund (UNFPA) sponsor *Twende na Wakati*. Since its inception, Population Communications International (PCI) has provided the technical assistance through their Nairobi office. Radio Tanzania, Dar es Salaam provides the technical staff and airs the program. When *Twende na Wakati* started to be aired in 1993 it was only broadcast on Radio Tanzania Dar es Salaam. Currently it is aired on other four different radio stations (Radio Tanzania - Dodoma, Sauti ya Tanzania - Zanzibar, Radio Faraja - Shinyanga and Sauti ya Injili - Kilimanjaro).

Twende na Wakati soap became an eye opener because in 1993/1994 another radio soap opera known as *Zinduka* (Wake up) was launched. The Reproductive and Child Health Section of the Ministry of Health with funding from the United States Agency for International Development (USAID) started the *Zinduka* radio soap. The technical assistance was provided by the Johns Hopkins University Center for Communication Programs. The objective of *Zinduka* is to "...promote quality reproductive and maternal health services" (Ministry of Health/RCHS 2001:2). Like *Twende na Wakati, Zinduka* is aired not only on Radio Tanzania Dar es Salaam but also on other radio stations like Radio Free Africa - Mwanza.

Apart from the two radio soaps that have been on air for almost a decade, many mini soaps have been broadcast in Tanzania since mid 1990s. In 1995, for example, the British Council in Dar es Salaam contracted Parapanda Arts Company to prepare a mini radio soap known as *Mnazi Mmoja*. The radio soap had thirty-two episodes that were broadcast on Radio Tanzania - Dar es Salaam. The objective of the radio soap was to provide voters' education to Tanzania prior to 1995 first general multiparty election.

In 1999 the Reproductive Health Unit – Ministry of Health, initiated another radio soap known as *Vijana Wetu*. It was a one-year weekly radio soap (52 episodes). The aim of *Vijana Wetu* was to provide adolescent reproductive health education to youth between 10 and 24 years of age. Parapanda Theatre also in 2000 secured funds from the Basket Fund and prepared a 24-episode radio soap known as *Bibi Msafiri* that was broadcast on Radio Tanzania – Dar es Salaam. The soap was on civic education.

Again in 2002, Parapanda Theatre was funded by Care International to produce a radio soap known as *Baragumu la Haki* (42 episodes). The aim of the radio soap was to provide civic education. *Baragumu la Haki* is still on air on Radio Tanzania – Dar es Salaam.

In 2003, a youth-based radio soap was sponsored by the African Youth Alliance (AYA). One of the objectives is to disseminate information on HIV/AIDS and Adolescent Reproductive Health. The radio soap 'Mambo Bomba' is broadcast by Radio Tanzania's Dar-es-Salaam; with technical support from PCI-Africa.

Why radio soaps in Tanzania? Almost all the monitoring and assessments done on the radio soap operas have come with positive findings. That is, radio soap operas are encouraging people to appreciate new behavior; are motivating them to seek out more information about how to adopt new behavior; and persuading them to become interested in practicing and advocating the new behavior as a norm for their society (Fossard 1998:7).

It is true that radio soap operas have a two- barrel gun that most of us believe helps the form to attain its objectives whenever it is implemented. First, the educational or cognitive component that radio soaps provide and how this helps people to change their attitudes towards certain things and practices. Second, is the element of entertainment that helps radio soaps to attract and retain more listeners throughout the life of the program.

The tradition of tale telling that is practiced in almost all Tanzanian communities has contributed to the success of radio soap operas in Tanzania. The nature of communication or the exchange of ideas in tale telling and in radio soap operas may be similar to other process of communication in which the communicator transfers a message to his/her listener. However, the additional factor of entertainment that the listeners/ audience experience provides the critical difference when compared with other channels of communication."

From his ten years of involvement in writing radio soap operas, Makoye said he had realized that this form (radio soap opera) is based on African tale telling techniques. Like in radio soap operas "…aesthetical experience in oral narrative-performance is made up of three inseparable components: captivation of audience, retention of audience and the transfer of cognitive experience to the audience. These three components are inseparable from each other in both radio soap operas and storytelling practices.

"In writing radio soap opera, a good story is very important. But what makes a good story? The patterning of episodes of the story is most important single factor in the attainment of the other two elements of aesthetic harmony: the emotive and cognitive satisfaction of the audience. In radio soap operas like in tale telling, for example, it is very important for a writer to relate images and actions in the story to a theme or a comment on a specific aspect of human behavior among the target audience. The actions or behaviors in the story must be capable of providing an overview about some of the recurrent concerns or values of the community.

Another factor that is highly employed in tale telling is the technique of elimination of boredom during the performance. This is done through the employment of other art forms like songs, dances, poems and so on. This technique is highly exploited in Tanzanian radio soap operas. In most radio soap operas, for example, there is tremendous use of songs, music, dances, recitations, drumming and so on. In actual fact, music has been a pivotal component in each episode. The use of these other art forms helps in manipulating listeners' emotions throughout the performance.

Another technique that is employed in both radio soap and storytelling is playing with the fluctuation of audience sensation. In both forms the technique is attempted through the paralleling together of two or more characters or stories that the audience is confronted with as an action progresses. In the long running radio soap opera *Twende na Wakati*, for example, one story started with two friends (Mkwaju and Shime). They were both employed as truck drivers and were staying in the same house. At the beginning they seemed to have the same characteristics. But when the story progresses they became two different persons. They developed different hobbies and aspirations that nobody amongst the audience expected. That made the story more catchy.

In both tale telling and radio soap operas, in order to engage the audience fully and ensure the appreciation of the message, the actions must be patterned in such a manner that they help to eliminate boredom by making the sensations of the audience fluctuate between activation and depression. In both forms, fluctuation of audience's sensations helps also to move the story forward. Moreover, it helps to create a cognitive focus for the audience vis-a-vis the characters' preoccupation.

Another technique mostly used in both tale telling and in radio soap operas is employment of characters and actions that help audience to identify themselves with whatever happens in the story. This technique also is highly used in most African narrative traditions.

In radio soap opera, character identification is the most crucial aspect in order to attain behavior change among listeners. Through character identification, "audience [listeners] find themselves loving some characters dearly, despising others, wanting to help those in need, and to like those they admire" (Fusser 1998:4).

Another important parallel technique that is highly employed in both tale telling and radio soap opera is audience participation. When discussing the aesthetic of oral narrative-performance in West Africa, Ruth Finnegan noted what she called audience behavior such as "spontaneous exclamations, actual questions . . . emotional reaction to the development of yet another parallel and repetitious episodes" (1977:232). In radio soap opera also audiences are highly encouraged to participate by using different means. For example, there are audiences who form discussion groups, others write or make phone calls to producers for further clarification or just to share their own experiences and understanding of the stories in the soap operas.

Finally, in most tell-tales the ending is always a happy ending. Likewise in radio soap operas especially the non-technical ones, the ending is always a happy one because the audience is always expected to have changed from negative to positive behavior."

Makoye concluded that the comparison between tale telling and radio soap operas techniques has shown that the radio soap opera, as a form of communication is not alien to Tanzanian audiences. It is gaining strong roots because it has a lot of aesthetic similarities with one of traditional and dearest art forms to the Tanzanian audiences which is the tale-telling tradition.

Things to ponder about:

- A concern was raised that it is difficult to get media owners who are perceived as obstacles, to participate in deliberations like the Soap Summit. It is important that they know the economic viability of these local programmes exists and that they support them in their Media Houses.

- Media liberalization has brought competition and as a result the struggle for audience competition. So the question of local programmes viability is not a problem that will last for a long time.

- In Nigeria, those producing soaps go to media houses and negotiate for partnerships, for example, for programmes to run for one year. They also agree that the stations can look for a sponsor for the soaps and whatever benefits are accrued, go to the station and not the producers of the soaps.

- Language needs to be accessible and there is a possibility that there is a disconnection between the writings coming out from writers and the 60% of audiences meant to receive but are not in this oral culture.

- The issue of conflict between donors and creative works is critical. Producers of soaps are forced to confine themselves to what the donors want and at times their creativity is stifled.

- The idea of using fables in entertainment and whether it has been effective needs to be investigated further.

IV

Social Change Programming

If entertainment-education is the process of purposely designing and implementing a media message to both entertain and educate, in order to increase audience members knowledge about an educational issue, create favourable attitudes, shift social norms and change overt behaviour as Singhal and Rogers (1999; 2002) have taught us, then it has a direct relationship to social change. Significantly, the aim of EE interventions is to contribute to planned and anticipated social transformation at the individual, community or societal levels. The social transformation may be made possible through an increase in levels of awareness and change of attitudes and positive behaviour. Audience members, for example, could adopt an HIV prevention behaviour as a result of the intervention. The EE strategy could also influence the external environment by helping create the necessary conditions for social change. It could contribute in social mobilization advocacy, and agenda-setting.

It is within this general purview, that a panel on social change programming was constituted at the Nairobi Soap Summit.

(The panelists included John Molefe of Soul City, South Africa; Holo Hachonda of ZIHP, Zambia; Michael Muindi, Kenya and Mumbi Kaigwa of the Theatre Company, Kenya. Herbert Makoye from Tanzania chaired this session.)

John Molefe of Soul City Institute of Health and Development Communication kicked off the session by presenting his paper on *"Social Change through the power of Mass Media"* in which he started by noting that media is not a magic bullet. It must be a part of a broader strategy for change. He continued to highlight some of the strategies that the Institute has used in their work. He reiterated that the media can be used to inform and raise awareness; create a supportive environment for change; stimulate open talk on issues such as sexuality, HIV and AIDS; to shift social norms; de- stigmatize; normalize safer sex, challenge attitudes and beliefs, connect people to help on the ground and advocate for policy action and accountability.

He then reported that according to research, edutainment programmes can be more effective and persuasive than conventional didactic programs that tell people how to behave. Entertainment broadcasting on radio and television reaches the largest audiences of any mass media programmes. Persuasive levels of the media are rated as follows: radio- 98%, television- 76% and print media as 55%. In his presentation Molefe pointed out that edu- tainment is useful due to its ability to persuade, inform, shift social norms and attitudes; stimulate dialogue and enhance horizontal communication and its commercial viability. Soul City has taken advantage of the usefulness of edu- tainment in its endeavor to educate its respective audience. Edu- tainement is a strategy based on a mixture of education and entertainment. It is accessible, popular and yet still serious enough to carry persuasive social messages.

In the communication initiatives Soul City has a prime time one hour long TV drama, a prime time radio drama broadcast in 9 African languages- which cover most of South Africa, three full color information booklets, which are distributed nationally through partner newspapers and non- governmental organizations. Soul City also uses the opportunity of the mass media to develop adult education and school life skills material and mount advocacy campaigns. This multi- media approach enhances message reception since each medium complements and reinforces the others.

Through this approach, the Institute has been able to carry a variety of topics including HIV/AIDS, youth sexuality, tobacco, tuberculosis, violence, hypertension, small business development, and violence against women in their series. In preparation of each series to ensure that the approach it takes and messages it sends out are accessible, relevant and clear, Soul City invests a lot in preparation of the series. This is particularly important in a context where health campaigns operate alongside advertising and commercial promotions that may be at odds with the health messages being sent out. Therefore, an advisory group is established for each issue to oversee the entire development process.

This group comprises of experts in media research, health promotion and adult education and social sciences. Literature review, audience research and wide consultations locally and internationally are undertaken to define the overall strategy. Available audience research is studied to identify major channels for communication and to inform the project of demographic profiles of prime time audiences for various channels. Before developing the messages, extensive research is conducted through focus groups with the audience in urban and rural areas to ascertain existing knowledge, attitudes and practices around the issues to be covered.

To establish the impact of Soul City on its audience, evaluation is conducted. Impact evaluation is done for every series. However, Soul City realizes that measuring the impact of a mass media communication vehicle is very difficult. Especially as behavior itself is complex and there are numerous influences on people's behavior, both positive and negative. Soul City evaluations are designed to deliberately engage with many of these measurement difficulties and attempted to document in great deal the extent to which the series succeeded or failed as a comprehensive health promotion intervention.

It was found that the reach and audience reception results show that Soul City is a popular edu-tainment vehicle with considerable reach across urban and rural populations of S. Africa. It competes favourably in the S. African media environment, highly valued by its target audience as relevant, credible and entertaining educational vehicle. It was also found to have played a significant role in social and behavior change in that it has increased awareness and accurate knowledge, stimulated interpersonal dialogue within families and other social networks, increased self-efficacy and a sense of empowerment (particularly among women), decreased experiences of negative social and peer pressure and in shifting people's attitudes, intentions and intermediate practice towards sustaining healthier behavior.

Soul City was also reported to have influenced positively the creation of a supportive environment for change in South Africa. This has been achieved through influencing people in leadership positions in communities, shapes, enhances and supplements communication between community leadership and their constituencies and begins the process of influencing reorientation of services. Furthermore, Soul City is reported to shift community norms, and to stimulate community dialogue and debate. It also increased access to service. The Stop Women Abuse Helpline helped to address a substantial need in the South African society, and increased access to crisis counseling and referral services for people affected by violence against women.

The Institute also runs a youth program *Soul Buddyz,* an edu-tainement vehicle, co- produced with SABC Education targeting children aged 8 to 12 years. The SABC through its department known as SABC Education, aims to educate children in an entertaining way. The SABC with its experience and expertise in the field of educational television is able to research, market and broadcast educational programs for children successfully.

Soul Buddyz consists of a 26 part television drama series, which was broadcast on SABCI (the largest South African public channel) at 18h30 weekly; a part 26 radio magazine series, piloted on three African language stations weekly for 30 minutes; a parenting booklet, 560 000 of which were distributed through newspapers nationally, and a grade 7 life skills book which was distributed through schools to grade 7 pupils nationally.

Soul Buddyz was broadcast first in August 2000. It dealt with issues such as children's rights, HIV/AIDS, youth sexuality, accidents, disability, road safety, gender equity and bullying. *Soul Buddyz* was developed in close consultation with the Department of Health and Department of Education and numerous NGO's working in the field.

An evaluation of *Soul Buddyz* was commissioned by the producers at the beginning of 2001. The evaluation consisted of a quantitative and a qualitative component, contracted separately to two independent research agencies, and coordinated by an independent researcher. The aim was to record the reach and audience reception of *Soul Buddyz* and to investigate the impact of *Soul Buddyz*- largely for the purpose of informing and improving subsequent series of *Soul Buddyz*. The evaluation looked at the impact of *Soul Buddyz* in the context of environmental factors, such as influences within families and the school environment. The results were then aired on television and booklets distributed.

It was found that *Soul Buddyz* seems to have had remarkably positive outcomes over the short term- both in terms of scope and depth of outcome. The popularity of the program observed in this evaluation are in many respects comparable to the impact of Soul City, the adult series. The fact that *Soul Buddyz* instantly compares so favorably with a well-established series may partially be due to the fact that the audience is young and relatively impressionable and therefore more receptive to media influences than older target audiences.

The observations on the work of Soul City can be a basis for future interventions in sub-Saharan Africa.

Holo Hachonda, the coordinator of the youth program at Zambia Integrated Health Program (ZIHP) talked about the lessons learned through the youth program. In his view, the youth understand best what their needs are and how they should be addressed. They can encourage their pees most effectively. By knowing what will have optimal impact, youth- led NGOs can catalyze young people in all areas, personally and programmatically. They also serve to advocate for youth- centered programs in government and other institutions.

According to Hachonda, ZIHP has four key interventions. These are; Youth Activists Organization (YAO), the Youth Media Group (YMG) Trendsetters, Africa Alive! And the HEART campaign.

The Youth Activists Organization (YAO)

YAO is a youth NGO formed in 1995 by high school graduates to address key civic, environmental, economic and health problems affecting Zambian Youth. It is supported by USAID, CEDPHA and JHU/CCP. The YAO has held a number of basic communications and facilitation skills training with the objective of equipping anti- AIDS clubs, religious and school youth leaders with better communication skills. So far YAO has been able to produce an inter- faith training curriculum *Treasuring the Gift*; train over 85 young people in schools, religious groups (Christian and Muslims) and youth clubs and reach over 300 youth directly. YAO also holds ARH (adolescence reproductive health) Soccer Camps with the objective of encouraging men to participate in sexual and reproductive health (SRH), HIV/AIDS, family planning (FP) and child health and other activities in the family. Their targeted audience include boys 14 to 24 years, in and out of school, both married and single. Primary school, secondary school students, parents of participants and community leaders. This intervention was implemented in nine districts: Chipata, Chongwe, Kafue, Nchelenge, Mpika, Lundazi, Kawambwa, Mwense and Mansa.

This initiative was also part of a collaborative Caring Understanding Partners (CUP) initiative, which included:- John Hopkins University Center for Communications Program, Society for Family Health (SFH), Zambia Information Services/ Population and Communication Project (ZIS/ POPCOM), Zambia Football Coaches Association (ZAFCA) and United States Peace Corps Volunteers (US-PCV). The activities of this intervention included SRH/HIV/ AIDS/ FP training for fathers and couples (JHU/CCP and SFH), coaches (YAO & ZAFCA), women (JHU/CCP, SFH, local health centers) and girls (YAO); Youth football skills (YAO, ZAFCA); Schools out reach sessions (YAO) and mobile video shows (SFH).

The Youth Media Group (YMG)

YMG is an organizations of young journalists established in *Trendsetters* in 1997. This organization targeted urban and peri- urban youth, in and out of school in its activities. YMG started with producing 500 copies of Trendsetters but the production went up to 32,000 copies per month at the moment. These copies include 12 000 for sale and 20,000 school edition copies. YMG also produces brochures for UNICEF and CCP on AIDS and contraceptives. *Trendsetters* is distributed in Lusaka and the Copper- belt region through schools and supermarkets. YMG has received two awards; *Global Media Award* from the Population Institute in 1997 and the *Millennium Pacesetters Award* from Radio Phoenix in 2000.

Africa Alive!

This is a bold multi- national, multi- media initiative using entertainment – education to improve ARH, reduce the spread of HIV/ AIDS/STDs among African Youth. Africa Alive has a number of activities that include; ICASA launch and concept September 1999 that included five ministers of health, an attendance of 5000 delegates and local youth and was broadcast on national TV for 2 hrs. *Africa Alive!* concerts were also held in Durban during the Durban 2000 AIDS conference in South Africa; *X-plosion* 2000 special is a 4 episode musical/ talk show on TV focusing on HIV/AIDS using popular musicians is developed through this group; 2000 Music festival that was held in July 2000; Alliance Francaise annual music day is organized by *Africa Alive!*; *Africa Alive!* also organizes World AIDS Day concerts; It sponsors the *Most Socially Conscious Artist Award* an annual *Ngoma Awards*; and also organizes HIV/AIDS youth rallies/ music concerts which are community and youth driven, have been held in seven communities and have reached 35, 000 directly and through these rallies launched *"Postcards and Pen pals"*.

The *HEART* Campaign

This is a national Youth Mass Media campaign that focuses on safer sex or abstinence for young people. It emphasis on leadership, full participation of young people in planning, designing, implementation, monitoring and evaluation. It also promotes positive peer pressure, changing community norms/ youth culture and youth supporting each other to practice abstinence or safer sex.

The target audience is segmented into males aged 14 to 19 years in the first phase of the program with the objective to encourage abstinence in this group. The slogan used was *"ili Che"* and through this abstinence is given a cool image. This program also aims at increasing consistence in condom use through the slogan " *You can't tell by looking"* and " *cool guys use condoms."*

Females aged 12- 19 years were also targeted with messages of abstinence *"Virgin Power, Virgin Pride"* was the slogan used. To encourage the consistent use of condoms among the sexually active adolescents the slogan used to target girls was *"Trust alone is not enough."*

The outcome of this campaign was five TV spots, five radio spots, three posters and notebooks. The campaign also produced car stickers and two music videos in the first phase. In phase two, the campaign produced five TV spots, 26 radio spots in seven languages, four posters, one music video and one music CD with all the songs produced on the campaign. In phase three, 5 TV spots-selected from Focus Group Discussions with audiences and stakeholders- resulted.

Partners in this project included youth NGOs acting as the advisory group; JHU/CCP; SFH; Central Board of Health; Network of People Living with HIV/AIDS; National HIV/AIDS/STD Council and Secretariat; Religious based organizations and networks and donors.

The program managed to reach 71% of urban youth and 37% of rural youth; substantially increased perceptions of risk; increased condom use at last sex vs. control group; increased communication about safe sex with partners and friends; increased abstinence among the study group vs. the control group and also increased self- efficacy of young women to refuse sex.

Holo Hachonda ended his presentation with recommendations that in order to make youth programs even more successful, youth need to strengthen their skills in management, budgeting, finance and report writing. This should be easy as youth are generally eager to learn. Youth also need financial resources and sustained emotional support to be successful. He also reiterated that youth- led efforts can translate into better youth-focused programming in both NGOs and government and must be promoted.

Michael Muindi of Research International gave a presentation on how *Ushikwapo Shikamana*, a Swahili radio soap opera produced by PCI and that has been broadcasting on Kenya Broadcasting Corporation (KBC) Radio since 1998, was designed. Muindi started his presentation by giving short background information on how the program began.

He explained that the current program was built on the success of an earlier program that was aired in the 1980s whose principle focus then was on reproductive health. Before the current program was created, formative research was conducted in 1998 to establish radio listenership reach and timings; family planning practices and general perceptions, maternal and child health issues, drug use and abuse practices, gender equity, HIV/AIDS awareness, adolescence sexual behaviour and social-cultural practices.

The methodology used to conduct this research was qualitative research. This involved Focus Group Discussions, in-depth interviews, and observations. A values grid was developed from the findings and content analysis which was done after four months to guide the script writers match educational issues to the program, generate cliff-hangers and emphasize the lessons to learn. Characters were developed to help pass the educational messages. The focus group discussions were composed of six to eight members. Male and female adults and male and female youth. The formative research was conducted in selected sites that is; Kibera slums in Nairobi, Kajiado which is rich in traditional culture, Machakos, which has the lowest fertility rates and Kisii, which has the highest fertility, rates in Kenya.

The Key findings were a high radio listenership among the study groups. The dominant broadcaster was KBC; the popular programs were those with educational and entertainment component; that youth tended to listen to programs with more music and drama content; that the youth were been drawn to the newer FM radio stations and that radios were easily affordable.

It was also clear that people needed to understand family planning (FP) well in order to remove suspicions from spouses of those using them, and men needed to be encouraged to be involved in FP decisions. It was found that despite the gains made in Maternal and child health there was still a lot to be done to eradicate the common diseases such as malaria, typhoid, respiratory tract infections, scabies, kwashiorkor, cholera among others.

It was also evident that there were increased incidences of adolescent sex due to peer pressure, poor or lack of parental guidance; inappropriate role models, unemployment and poverty. Drug use and abuse was on the increase. It was claimed that drug use was on the rise because people used them in order to cope with the day to day problems and pressures of life, to feel good and happy, to gain strength and knowledge, to escape reality, stay awake and to keep away diseases. It was evident that the main substances of abuse were heroin, bhang and khat.

It was found that HIV/AIDS infection rates were going up despite increased awareness of the AIDS fatality. It was also clear from the findings that denial of its existence was a major problem in some areas. Gender played a big role in the HIV/AIDS pandemic. There was mutual-gender- wise suspicion of infection source. It was felt by the study population that the main source of transmission was sexual intercourse. It was discovered that people knew that the only ways to prevent infection from HIV was through protection (ABC of HIV), which are abstinence, behavior change and consistent condom use. However it was felt that there is a problem with the protection because people abscond from safe sexual practices due to lack of correct and adequate information, fatalism, rape, and cultural practices such as female genital cut.

FGC was found to be sporadic in some parts of the study areas. This is because this practice is highly valued as a rite of passage into adulthood, it is reported to restrain female sexuality, which was seen as good, and their communities have accepted its propagation.

Monitoring and Evaluation

The program is evaluated and monitored quarterly. The objective is to monitor and evaluate the program listenership; to provide feedback from the listeners to script writers and incorporate any emerging issues, to make program more interactive and people friendly and to ensure audience ownership of the program. Over the years the feedback that monitoring has elicited has influenced the direction of the program. Issues that have been dealt with due to audience feedback include fertility and family planning, STD, maternal and child health, socio- cultural issues such as gender equity and equality, and economic issues.

Different sites have been visited for monitoring all over the country and these include Nairobi's Kibera, Kangemi, Ongata Rongai and Pumwani areas; Voi; Machakos; Nakuru; Kerugoya; Kajiado; Kericho; The rural areas include Kutus, Mwatate, Kangundo/ Matungulu and Londiani. The multiplicity of areas have helped to gather varying views, opinions and perceptions about the program leading to overall improvement over the years. The methodology used is qualitative research and included focus group discussion, in- depth interviews and observations. It has been found that HIV/AIDS knowledge is high, that institutions to deal with the scourge in rural areas are scarce moreover they are ill equipped, understaffed. Social stigma is high though declining slowly. The spread of HIV is mainly propagated by harmful cultural practices mentioned above.

Through the years, stakeholders have been able to pass important health promotion and social change messages through *Ushikwapo Shikamana* Program. These include the fact that everyone is at risk of HIV infections but that HIV infection can be avoided. Through the program writers have also dealt with issues such as the need for care of HIV/AIDS infected and affected persons; stigma; orphans; corruption; environment; drug use and abuse; women's empowerment; eradication of female circumcision; family planning and male involvement; and child's rights. The program came to an end in June 2004, after five and a half years of Broadcast. 576 new episodes went on air through the Kenya Broadcasting Corporation.

Mumbi Kaigwa made a presentation titled *Making TV and Film in Kenya: The Case of Heart and Soul.*

She began by pointing out that in the last ten years, there has been an increase in the desire to make local programmes and films using home grown talent, as opposed to the more traditional use of Kenya as a location with a few jobs for the local film crews and African actors providing colour in supporting secondary roles. This kind of work has the potential of bringing the strongest social message of all– the message of pride and a sense of belonging. Using the power of imagination, television and radio can create fictional scenarios that tie us to a changing present. We are no longer bound in the past; we are no longer unable to see ourselves in the future. Images of ourselves with an ability to talk, laugh, to dream, a vision of a future that we can create.

Mumbi pointed out that Kenyans have not made many films but *Kolormask, Kitchen Toto, Saikati 1 and 2,* as well as the recent video *Dangerous Affairs* have been enthusiastically received by a public hungry for their own stories. *Heart and Soul* sought to capitalise on this success, with Kenyans in lead acting and technical roles, telling contemporary African stories and using the medium in a professional manner while at the same time, using drama as a teacher. Anecdotal evidence as well as formal research carried out at the end of the broadcast run demonstrates that the show is on the right path.

Heart and Soul was born out of the success of two music videos that were produced by the UN-Drug Control Programme, to commemorate the International Day Against Drug Abuse in 1994 and 1995. Documentation was available to show that the soap opera genre had been used for social marketing in countries with similar concerns as our own. Stories about success in South Africa, Philippines and Mexico were particularly encouraging. However it wasn't until March 2000 and after much discussion with various UN agencies including the UN Information Center that 24 information officers met to discuss how soap operas could be used to give a human face to the UN mandate.

Soon after, and after failed attempts to source technical assistance from the makers of South Africa's *Soul City*, a relationship was struck with producer and directors from the BBC soap opera *Eastenders*. Four Kenyan writers were chosen as story liners and together with 12 other writers participated at an initial writers workshop with a producer and a storyliner from BBC. The storyliners spent three days initially building the characters complete with their comprehensive back-stories as well as the broad outlines for stories of 26 episodes. Other experts would join later development stages to give workshops in acting and directing for the camera.

After the workshop, which produced a draft of the first two episodes, six writers were chosen from the sixteen workshop participants to write the remaining four episodes of the initial six-part pilot. At the time, the intention was that the remaining ten writers might be called upon to provide a pool of writers for the second series. In fact, this was the thinking behind all the training for writers, directors and actors. Anyone who had gone through the initial training sessions might be called upon to audition for subsequent roles in the series. It was the intention of the project to provide training for as many actors as possible even if they never got a part on *Heart and Soul*.

The series was broadcast in July 2002 on KBC TV and radio and through the satellite channel TV Africa, to Kenya and 11 other African countries. It was repeated in Kenya in December of the same year. During the period between this first workshop and the televised broadcast, fundraising continued and interested parties from the UN, various departments of the Kenyan government and from the private sector made this project the first to bring together a large number of the UN family, the private sector and diverse government agencies in a joint project. Fund raising for the project's second series is currently on going under a steering committee headed by the UN Information Center and the budget has been reworked to provide for the following four main outputs:

- Fundraising, distribution and promotion
- Management, legal, finance and administration systems.
- Communication and media strategy development
- Creative development and production.

The six episodes of the TV version were broadcast over a four-week period. The programme explores a range of social economic and development issues such as HIV/AIDS, poverty eradication and gender issues. It also deals with the issue of family conflict.

Consumer Insight, a local research company carried out a quantitative research to determine the successes and shortcomings of the programme. This information will assist in the development of a new series. The research company was asked to determine the profile of programme viewers and listeners, to gather audience reactions to programme settings, characters and storylines, and to evaluate the programme's communication effect.

Respondents to the questionnaires were asked a series of questions to determine viewing habits their preference between this and other soap operas both local and foreign.

Mumbi Kaigwa emphasized:

"If we were to start over again, and I do hope that the various interested parties will find the approximately $ 1.9 million that has been budgeted to complete the next 26 episodes, I would hope that a strong sense of ownership was clearer in all sectors- from donors to the creative and particularly the media which has been scathing in its criticism about the amounts of money being spent to produce feature films and programmes for TV, which is unfortunate as there is lack of adequate background. One often feels that those who could have played a stronger role in sharing the facts have ignored the opportunities presented and neglected their duty to do so."

"I don't have to tell those of you who are making local television programmes just how difficult the road is that we have chosen to travel. I've heard it said that there is no need for the amount of technical tweaking and professionalism that *Heart and Soul* attempted to deliver as:

a) Kenyans want to watch foreign films and TV programmes;
b) There are foreign TV programmes which can be purchased for very little money, and
c) Local viewers are watching the local programmes with little or no complaint so why bother?"

However, taken with a long-term view, and with relevant inputs, at least in the case of Kenya, the price making local programmes will come down."

According to Mumbi Kaigwa, *Heart and Soul* is just one programme of what should be many and one of the problems of the *Heart and Soul* project was the lack of adequate and focussed public relations. There are so few benchmarks for contemporary Kenyan stories told in English and therefore this made the programme be picked for all the wrong reasons.

Heart and Soul is important in very many ways. Most importantly, is the way it begins. It gives a sense of dignity and hope to a continent which has been much aligned; demonstrates that the art of passing on life's valuable lessons through story telling is not dead and that the stories that Africans have told for centuries do have a place in the modern world.

Things to ponder about:

- There is need to use available resources to produce local programmes. It is also important for film and video producers to network among themselves and other artists. We should also look at social programmes cutting across the social spectrum.

- The question of sustainability and what mechanisms are in place once the donors pull out arose. South Africa has a history of very strong civil society (CSOs). The CSOs have been pressuring the public broadcaster to have a quota for local programmes. Local programmes are also being supported to be of quality so that they can attract advertisers. Income comes from commercial sector for *Soul City* programmes. The organization also gets money from the Public Broadcaster since programmes are produced independently. Productions are done in all languages of South Africa and also work in partnership with others.

- The lifestyles of slum dwellers are lacking in many media work. Producers should focus on these people.

- *Soul City* has productions with perspectives from the informal settlings and rural areas. But the challenge for *Soul City* is to have something aspirational for the diverse audiences of South Africa.

- There are great programmes coming from Africa. But how do we monitor behaviour change as opposed to creating awareness?

- Producers should not be deterred by criticism particularly if they are focused on making positive changes as opposed to making money. They should realize that most people find it very easy to criticize.

The issues raised by the various panels are pertinent. By focussing on them, we may be able to chart a path through which we can deal with the burning issues of the day – HIV prevention, care and treatment of HIV positive people, social support, the fate of children orphaned by children, destigmatization and acceptance as well as the place of power in sexual relations.

V

Numerous radio soap operas have emerged in Africa since mid 1980s when Kenya launched the first ever long range soap opera on health through the then Voice of Kenya. The experience gained by the production team in putting together Ushikwapo Shikamana opened avenues for the growth of the genre in East Africa. Also a follow up soap was designed in mid 1990s. Some of the writers, producers and artists involved in the Ushikwapo of the 1980s were to play a central role in the sequel.

In the following contribution, put together by a team of young researchers based in Nairobi, and who have been closely associated with the program under a PCI-Africa mentoring program, we hear the voices of the youth as they interpret the Kenyan radio soap opera. The contribution is reproduced in its entirety in order to capture the essence of this important health related radio program.

Ushikwapo Shikamana: Increasing Dialogue in Communities

Mary Kabura, Lucy Muriithi & George Gathigi

An extract from *Ushikwapo Shikamana*:

(Ulimboni City. Sineno visits her lover Haiba at his residence. Slow music can be heard faintly. Other natural sounds like birds singing, cock crowing can be heard intermittently)

Sineno:	Darling, you really made me anxious when you left a message urging me to see you urgently.
Haiba:	It is very important and urgent. I tried calling you on your cellphone without success. That is why I left you the message.
Sineno:	Oh yah! I gave the driver to recharge it in the office.
Haiba:	That is ok. I really wanted to see you.
Sineno:	Go on here I am, my love.

Haiba:	Hold on. Just relax. Open this bottle of wine and take a drink as we talk.
Sineno:	*(Anxiously)* Mmh! What is wrong? It is not like you to be generous with your wine stock. You would rather go out and buy one so as to save your precious stock!
Haiba:	No sweat, there is always something new in this world.
Sineno:	Just as I was to you
Haiba:	All new things are welcome until their novelty wears off.
Sineno:	*(laughs)* don't start your wise-cracks.. You really amuse me *(Laughs)*
Haiba:	Laughter is the best panacea for thoughts, loneliness and low mood swings. It enhances your self image and confidence and makes one feel up to facing the world.
Sineno:	Thank you; but what do you mean? Are you still hunting? Looking for something younger? Better?
Haiba:	I am not in the market anymore. Not now; not for ever. I gave up the hunting game along time ago.
Sineno:	*(sighs)* Aah. You of all people! Take care lest what you wish for becomes real!
Haiba:	Go on dreaming. You will have a long wait. There is an end to everything and this is where the buck stops.
Sineno:	I don't understand you, dear. What do you mean?
Haiba:	You will definitely understand after I tell you why I needed to see urgently.
Sineno:	*(anxiously)* Are you trying to tell me that our relationship is over?
Haiba:	Not my words… Maybe if that is what you want.
Sineno:	Reason?
Haiba:	My next question exactly *(silence)*. There is a beginning and an end to everything. However, the end to our relationship is not welcome. It is being forced on us.
Sineno:	I knew this would happen. My fears and anxieties have materialised! You really cheated me into being your lover and

	after giving you my body, my love, my everything you discard me?
Haiba:	That is not my aim and I didn't really want this to happen. It just happened. I am not in control any more.
Sineno:	That is not true… I will not waste more time listening to more lies. Goodbye, Haiba.
Haiba:	Just a minute… I still love you more than anything else, Sineno, but our future depends on what you decide.
Sineno:	What I decide?
Haiba:	Yes, over what I am going to tell you.
Sineno:	Go ahead. I am all ears.
Haiba:	Do you remember last time we were together when I told you that I was going to see a doctor?
Sineno:	Yes I do.
Haiba:	The examination results were very distrurbing.
Sineno:	In what way?
Haiba:	It was revealed that I have HIV; that is, I am HIV positive.
Sineno:	*(A glass shutters. Silence)* What! Oh my God… you mean you have AIDS Haiba?
Haiba:	Not yet. I don't have AIDS; but I am HIV positive.
Sineno:	*(Tearfully)* Why didn't you tell me before? You must have infected me! Oh my God… *(Cries desperately)*
Haiba:	Crying will not solve anything, darling. You need to be examined to determine your status.
Sineno:	*(Cries intensely)* what stupidity led me into having unprotected sex? Haiba… why have you killed me…? Oh God what shall I do?…

Background

Ushikwapo Shikamana was first broadcast in 1987 to 1989 and was designed to tackle issues of family planning and was funded by the *National Council of Population and Development* (NCPD) and produced by

Tom Kazungu of the Kenya Broadcasting Corporation (the then Voice of Kenya). The soap opera was designed to motivate listeners to adopt family planning methods. The program grew out of a 1983 workshop on entertainment-education soap opera design in Mexico organized by Population Communications International (PCI), an NGO involved in soap operas for social change and family planning (Singhal & Rogers 1999: 130).

The program won the 1989 Global Award in Media Excellence as the Best Radio Program in Population Reporting, its sequel went on to win this award in 2001. The intervention was a thirty minute twice a week (with two reruns) radio soap opera on family harmony. The program contributed in increasing the numbers of new users of family planning methods and lowered fertility rates nationally, according to research findings (Mazrui et al, 1989, Ochillo, 1989).

Ushikwapo was designed and written using modeling of behaviors as its centrepiece. Further creative strategies relating to the development of characters and the use of the multiplots utilized effectively, by drawing on melodrama. Formative research carried out before scripting the episodes contributed greatly to the richness and authenticity of the drama.

In November 1998, PCI with support from the Ford Foundation launched *Ushikwapo Shikamana 2* (If Assisted, Assist Yourself), a fifteen-minute sequel of *Ushikwapo Shikamana 1*. The soap is supported by a comic strip, which appeared three times a week on TAIFA LEO, Kenya's national Kiswahili Daily since December 22, 1999 to December 2003.

Synopsis

Ushikwapo Shikamana 2 is set in three locations: Kanyageni which is a slum and peri- urban characterised by non- formal settlements and poor environmental conditions, Langoni is a rural setting characterised by traditional practices and Ulimboni an urban and affluent is everybody's' dream home. Each of these locations presents different problems and issues. There are three main characters: positive, transitional and negative characters.

Tatu, for instance, a teacher is the main positive character, providing a vehicle and a model for directed positive change. She practices family planning and fights against early and forced marriages. Shindo, on the other hand is a negative role model - rich, corrupt, and uncouth. In the course of the drama, the positive characters are rewarded, the transitional helped to become positive and the negative punished for their antisocial ways.

In 1998, the first year of broadcast, *Ushikwapo Shikamana* went on air at 6:00 p.m. –6:15 pm (Mondays and Wednesdays) and 2:30-3:00 p.m. (Saturdays). Due to a major power rationing that affected the country, Kenya Broadcasting Corporation (KBC) shifted the program to a time that electricity was available following PCI's persuasion. Thus going on air at peak time at no extra charge in the second half of the second year. The radio soap broadcasts on the Kiswahili Station of KBC twice a week on Mondays and Wednesdays with a 30-minute omnibus on Saturdays. It goes on air at Peak Time (Super "A" Time) – 8:45 p.m. – 9:00 a.m. on Mondays and Wednesdays, and "C" Time on Saturdays – 2:30 – 3:00 p.m. Having the radio program on air at super A time presents a major opportunity of capturing majority of listeners in the family units. The language of the soap is Kiswahili, Kenyan's national language.

In consecutive years of broadcast, the program has retained the peak time, with a small discount from KBC, as the drama is socially committed. *Ushikwapo Shikamana* has been rated as the number one drama program on KBC According to a 1998 evaluation of Ushikwapo Shikamana estimated a regular audience of 7 million people, 40% of Kenya's population (Singhal & Rogers, 1999: 130). The program is written by: Kimani Njogu (Head Scriptwriter), Juma Mrisho, Lolani Kalu and Scholastica Waweru and is produced by Tom Kazungu at the Apex Productions studios.

The radio program transmits its messages in a drama form based on themes and issues experienced by ordinary Kenyans in their day-to-day lives. These themes/issues include: cultural practices such as female genital cut (FGC), early marriages, traditional gender roles of men and women, domestic violence, income generating activities, modern marriages, drug abuse, reproductive and sexual health, family planning and maternal and child health, spousal communications, modeling, and STIs/HIV/AIDS among others.

Prior to the program development, an elaborate formative research was carried out in 1998 and some of the issues addressed in the 1980s revisited. The sites for the formative research were Kajiado, Machakos, Kibera and Kisii. Kajiado is reported to have deep- rooted cultural and traditional practices such as FGC; early and forced marriages for girls and boy to girl child preferences. Machakos was selected for its low fertility rates despite high sexual activity and the onset of sexual activity at early age in the population. It also has a rural setting. Kibera was selected because of its diversity in cultures, high prevalence of HIV infection and high levels of poverty. On the other hand Kisii was selected due to the fact that there are high fertility rates among the people and also a prevalence of harmful cultural practices like FGC.

Nonetheless new issues were incorporated into the drama (Kimani Njogu, 2000). An independent research team conducted a situational analysis that would inform the issues to be covered and emphasized through the program. As a result of the formative research, a range of seven broad issues were identified and integrated into a framework of educational issues and a values grid. Specifically;

(a) Reproductive health issues to include; fertility values and family planning
(b) Maternal and child health issues and values
(c) Sexual health issues to include sexually transmitted infections (STIs) and HIV/AIDS
(d) Gender Issues
(e) Social cultural issues and values
(f) Economic issues and values.

These issues formed the basis on which education was to be carried out. Each of these issues and values was then broken down into smaller statements in a tabular format indicating in one column the educational issue, then a positive statement about it and, in the third column, a negative one. For example, with respect to social/cultural issues and values we have eleven educational issues.

Below is an example of one educational issue:

Sexually Transmitted Infections Issues and Values

Educational Issues	Positive values (It is good that...)	Negative values (It is bad that...)
1. People do not understand that the major risk factors for HIV/AIDS and other STD's are (1) promiscuity, (2) unprotected sex with an infected persons, (3) sex with male or female sex commercial workers, (4) unsafe sexual practices, and (5) sharing of razors and needles.	...people understand the major risk factors for contracting HIV/AIDS are having multiple partners, having unprotected sex with female and male commercial sex workers, not using condoms, and sharing razors and needles.	...people do not understand the major risk factors for AIDS, and wrongly believe that AIDS is spread by (1) condoms (2) hugging/kissing, (3) insects, and (4) caring for an AIDS patient.
2. People do not understand that there are means to protect themselves from getting AIDS/HIV and other STD's.	...people understand the major risk factors for contracting HIV/AIDS and other STD's by (1) practicing abstinence, (2) practicing mutual monogamy, (3) using condoms, and (4) not sharing razors/needles.	...people wrongly believe that there are means to protect themselves from getting HIV/AIDS and other STD's.
3. People believe that HIV/AIDS is not always fatal or that there is a cure for it.	...people understand that HIV/AIDS is a fatal disease for which there is no cure.	...people believe that AIDS is a curable or non-fatal disease.
4. People believe that AIDS only affects certain groups of people (e.g.. certain races, certain age groups, only skinny people, etc.)	...people understand that the HIV/AIDS virus can infect them if they engage in high risk behaviour.	...people do not understand that AIDS can infect them if they engage in risky behaviour.

5. People believe that they can tell who has the HIV virus by looking at them, by judging their character, or some other unreliable means.	...people understand that healthy-looking people can have the HIV virus and that only a blood test can determine whether someone has HIV.	...people wrongly believe that they can judge who has HIV and who does not based on unreliable means.
6. People do not understand the importance of using condoms as a reliable means of protection against HIV/AIDS and other STD's.	...people understand that by using condoms correctly they can protect themselves from AIDS and other STD's.	...People do not understand that condoms are ineffective protection from AIDS and other STD's, or believe condoms spread AIDS.
7. People believe that HIV/AIDS tests are for pregnant women, prostitutes, and STD/AIDS patients.	...people understand that HIV/AIDS tests are available to the general public, but only at all major hospitals.	...people misunderstand that HIV/AIDS tests are available only for certain groups.
8. People do not understand that even if they are monogamous they can get AIDS if their spouse/partner has other sexual partners.	...people understand that even if they are monogamous they can get AIDS if their spouse/partner has other sexual partners.	..people do not understand even if they are monogamous they can get AIDS if their spouse/partner has other sexual partners.
9. People do not seek proper treatment for STI's.	..people seek medical treatment for STI's.	..people are not treated, or seek traditional treatment, for STI's.
10. Men believe that they will not get AIDS if they only have sex with young girls and virgins thereby increasing both their own and their partner's risk of contracting HIV/AIDS.	...men understand that they can contract HIV from any infected person and they can transmit to any other person(young girls or virgins).	...men act as "sugar-daddies" and put themselves and their partners at risk of HIV/AIDS.

Issues Covered During The Course of the Program: Over the years the program has been instrumental in educating its audience on a number of issues that include;

Ideal families: Through a dramatic examination of the Shindo-Maua/ Jaka- Tatu marriages, listeners were invited to evaluate their lives and what it would take to improve the quality of family life. Other marriages that are scrutinized are those of Gogo–Chezi and Mchikichi-Shikalao.

Shindo is a greedy, promiscuous, corrupt and self-confessed male chauvinist. Despite his vast wealth he does not seem to get enough. He is a negative role model from Ulimboni and runs a drugs syndicate in town, has a big supermarket in town and uses his money to lure girls into his trap. Shindo has no respect for his wife Maua. Shindo hates that his wife Maua has not borne him a son. He needs a boy to inherit his vast wealth. Thus he decides to take a second wife, Chausiku, an employee at one of his supermarkets. Chausiku bears him a son. His promiscuous behaviour however ultimately lands Shindo in trouble with Maua. She divorces him. Meanwhile, Shindo is having problems with the law due to his drug dealings. Shindo's violent behaviour towards his wife (Maua) lands him in prison.

On the other hand, Jaka is the exact opposite of Shindo in that he is caring and loving to his wife Tatu. He also promotes dialogue in his family setting which encourages his wife to greater heights of human rights activism and community development at Kanyageni. She is an important role model to girls and women in her community.

Traditional cultural practices: These are reflected in the program in terms of FGC, forced marriages and preference for the boy child. Cultural practices detrimental to health, which include female genital cut (FGC) and early and forced marriages are discussed at length. Through the experiences of Pendo who suffers physically and psychologically after being subjected to the rite, the audience is invited to re-examine the practice and to reject it. On being circumcised and forced into marrying an old man (Mzee Konga), Pendo runs away into the city (Ulimboni) where she is employed as house help by Maua, Shindo's wife.

However, Shindo, a big time womanizer entices the girl with gifts and money. Pendo feels attracted to Shindo because he is the only person who seems to understand her and to love her as a person; a love denied by her parents who forcefully circumcised her and almost had her married. As the story unfolds she loses her job when Maua suspects that she is having an affair with her husband Shindo. Shindo buys her a house because he "cares and would not want her to suffer". Unwittingly, she gives in to take some alcoholic drinks and in her drunken mode, has sex with him for the first time.

Pendo blames her parents for not giving her the opportunity of continuing with education and instead forcing her into circumcision and marriage. Her mother seeks forgiveness, but Pendo is not very forgiving. Meanwhile, she finds her love in Sulubu, a younger man who is attracted to her. But she must disconnect with Shindo before she can start a relationship with Sulubu.

Gogo, a conservative traditional man believes that women are inferior and nothing good can come of listening to them. He is abusive to his wife – Chezi – and forces his son, Kinga into marriage. Kinga refuses and runs into a peri-urban area (Kanyageni) to start a new life away from the conservatism of his father. When Kinga falls in love with Lulu-an urban well-behaved girl- and wants to marry her, his father is opposed to the marriage because (i) she is uncircumcised (ii) she is not from his village. But the young people love each other. Eventually, a marriage based on love and mutual understanding other that ethnicity, origin, or subscription to a cultural practice is presented as the more viable solution. Through the determination of Kinga and Lulu, and the support mechanisms that they have put in place, Gogo reluctantly allows the marriage to take place.

HIV/AIDS: The incidence of HIV/AIDS in Kenya is frightening. In the drama, we see people dying and being buried in thousands. At certain moments, there are those who argue that there is no disease that has no cure. They try traditional medicine and when this fails, excuses such as that the disease was too advanced, are sought. "If only the person had visited the medicineman before he was overcome by the disease..." they mutter. But people continue dying. "What type of disease is this?" people ask. All sorts of rumors associated with HIV/AIDS are discounted. Listeners receive information on behavior that puts one at the risk of contracting HIV/AIDS. The difference between HIV/ and full-blown AIDS is elucidated, as well as issues of stigma, treatment and support.

Dialogue in the family: Most spouses hardly talk about sexual and reproductive health issues. Decision making on matters affecting the family is almost always viewed as a domain restricted to the man. Women are hardly involved. Through the interaction between Jaka and Tatu before and after marriage, it is evident that an alternative behavior, in which decision making is shared, is preferred. Jaka and Tatu are presented as models of the ideal husband and wife. Before they get married, the two are engaged in major negotiations. Tatu does not want to leave her rural school when she gets married. Instead she would like Jaka to join her there and this Jaka finds difficult: culturally, women join women and not the other way. Why should his marriage to Tatu be an exception? After intense discussions with Lulu, Kinga, Maua and other individuals, he accepts her request to move when they eventually get married. Furthermore, they agree that they will only have two children of whichever gender reflecting the underlying issue of child spacing and rights of women over their bodies, which can only succeed if both partners are equal stakeholders in the process of decision making.

Drug Use and Abuse: Shindo is involved in a very lucrative business in drugs. This is a full fledged industry, for which he has employed a team of boys facing economic hardships as "workers." They include Nyundo (the Hammer), who later becomes their leader. Nyundo is the only one of the gang members who is directly answerable to Shindo himself; and, as such, they forge a very close crooked relationship. Later Nyundo's position is challenged by Pangupangu, Kinga's younger brother.

There are clashes over territory. Carlos, a leader of one of the gangs is liquidated by Nyundo. Carlos' death, nevertheless, fails to bring a much longed for sigh of relief to Shindo and his henchmen; because his number two, Noriega, takes over the gang and provides a real challenge to Shindo.

In order to broaden the market of their illegal trade, Shindo, Nyundo, Pangupangu, and Noriega target the streets and educational institutions for their activities. Through dramatic twists, the practice of drug use and abuse is exposed. Model police officers, exemplified by Inspector Kato, are presented as crucial for the eradication of drug related crimes. Kato is contrasted with Inspector Tonge, a corrupt officer who works in cohorts with Shindo and other criminals. Mabuche is a drug addict. He is involved in petty crime in order to buy drugs. By the end of the second year of broadcasts, the young man is shown as fully dependent on drugs supplied to him occasionally by Pangupangu, Kinga's brother. Through the efforts of Zawadi (Mabuche's sister who runs away from her home in order not to be circumcised), Kinga, Tatu, and Jaka Mabuche is later rehabilitated and involved in the anti drug campaign.

This issue is dealt with in detail as it has plagued the Kenyan youth whose very lives are destroyed by drugs and alcohol with increasing intensity.

Gender violence and son preference: This is mainly dealt with through an examination of the Shindo-Maua marriage. Shindo is a violent and abusive husband. He has extra-marital relationships with many women, which puts him at risk of being infected with STIs/HIV/AIDS and re-infecting his wife. On one occasion, he infects her with an STI and she is a very worried woman. When he beats her so that she miscarries a child he believes is a girl, she deserts him. Maua works closely with Lulu, a positive character in the drama to come to terms with her situation. Issues of psychological violence, FGC and rape are discussed.

Family Planning and Maternal-Child Health: Different methods of family planning are presented through Maua, Chausiku, Tatu-Jaka and Kinga-Lulu. Unwanted and unplanned pregnancies that may result in unsafe abortion especially among teenagers is shown as the failure to use contraceptives. Through the characters the different forms of contraceptives and family planning methods are discusses.

Magimagi, an adolescent girl has a sexual relationship with the sweet talking Pangupangu. Unknown to Magimagi, he is also having a relationship with Chaku, her mother. Separately and for different reasons, Chaku and Pangupangu would like Magimagi to abort. However, the girl knowing the consequences of abortion is hesitant and unwilling. Eventually, she decides to carry the pregnancy and bring up her child.

Community Empowerment: Collective community development and mobilizing for change by the rural women (such as Chezi and Shikalao) under the guidance of Tatu is shown as the most viable way of ensuring the empowerment of women. For instance, Maua is initially dependent on Shindo and consequently stays in an abusive relationship. However, through her interaction with Lulu – the hair stylist- she sets up her own business and is able to separate from her abusive husband. Thus she paves the way for her own growth and for the collapse of her husband who lives dangerously.

Girls opposed to female circumcision (such as Zawadi) are assisted by the local primary school teacher Tatu (a major change agent in the community) and older women who have transformed their attitudes and behavior in the course of the drama to run away from their village to a school in Kanyageni. Here they are enrolled and given an opportunity to continue with their education. This has been modeled after the AIC Kajiado school which hosts girls who flee FGC and forced marriages in their communities.

Pambo, Lulu's niece, seeks a non-conventional career. She is a first class artist and model. But most people are opposed to her strong urge to pursue modeling. Nonetheless, she provides a series of examples of women who are morally upright and beautiful. Moreover, she argues that there is nothing inherently wrong or immoral in modeling and believes success is eminent. Despite opposition from her family to this career they eventually come to respect the decision. Pambo's physical beauty endears her to men. Haiba, Bahati's lover, finds her irresistible but when he makes a move, he is quickly repulsed. Shindo hopes that he can win her over. But the girl is too empowered as a result of her interaction with Lulu, a positive role model, to be manipulated.

The values' grid developed at the Ushikwapo Shikamana design workshop has continued to guide the scriptwriting process. The script content analysis shows the consistency with which educational messages are interwoven in the story.

Research and Monitoring

Monitoring is critical to the program's sustainability and success. It serves to confirm that the program is achieving its objectives in reaching its intended audiences with educative messages and that the messages are beneficial to the audience. *Ushikwapo Shikamana* has been monitored from its inception by independent researchers who carry out the monitoring and evaluation of the program on a quarterly basis.

Monitoring is carried out as field visits to selected areas to collect feedback on the program through focus group discussions. They also review and analyze letters from listeners; listen to and monitor the messages in the program related to the values grid. Subsequently, they also meet with the creative and production teams regularly to share the responses from the field. However, this activity that is carried out consequently with the airing of the program. Equally, the comic strip is subjected to values' grid analysis, which gives us an idea of what has been covered.

Although a number of private radio stations have recently started broadcasting in Kenya, *Ushikwapo Shikamana* has continued going on air through the national service of Kenya Broadcasting Corporation (KBC). The choice results from our recognition that KBC has a regional listener ship in East Africa. Research has shown that 99% of all the people who listen to the radio regularly, listen to the KBC and of these 70% listen to KBC Kiswahili service. Furthermore, the fact that the program is aired at Super A Time gives it the opportunity of capturing a significant slice of that listener ship.

After the first year of broadcast, epilogues were introduced and used regularly not only to heighten the drama but also to call on the audience to take concrete steps to deal with the issues raised in the drama. The introduction of a referral system into the program through the provision of information of where the audience can access specific services has acted as a motivation to the audience. Through the availing of a list of relevant organizations, their contact information with their approval on air audience members have been empowered to be actively involved in effecting change in their societies.

Listener groups and clubs were also formed in a quest to involve the audience in the development of the program. By asking the audience to write about what they found useful about the program; issues they would like tackled in the program have continually been able to give the audience ownership to the program. In effect we have received letters of people whose lives have been positively affected by the program, some claiming to have been saved from eventual demise.

Sample Letters

"I would like to give my views on the program, Ushikwapo Shikamana.

First, I am thirty years old, married and I have four children.

My husband has been mistreating me by assaulting me. The children have also been suffering. They even sleep hungry. When he comes home at night he is always drunk. He starts beating the children with no reason and when I dare ask him, he turns on me. He even locks us outside to spend the night in the cold.

One day I convinced him and we listened to the program on the radio called Ushikwapo Shikamana. We got good teachings on how we can live well, understanding each other and taking care of the family.

From that day we listened to the program, we have been blessed together; he has changed and has become a very good person. Therefore I would like to thank all those who are concerned for presenting this play".

(Agripinah Njeri Alila)

"Receive my greetings and gratitude for the program that educates and entertains. I would like to give my thanks to Kinga and Lulu. To Lulu; for being patient and continued love for the husband even after being told of his fertility problems. Because many of the women today could not hold on and they would have left Kinga. This is a big lesson to women and girls who are married or are hoping to get married.

I would like to give you one case. There is a man from my area who married a very beautiful girl. After marriage they stayed for eight years without succeeding in getting a child. They started blaming each other and later separated for nine years.

But from the advice of Kinga and Lulu, when they heard that Kinga could now make his wife pregnant after seeing the doctor, they realized that even men could have fertility problems. After listening to the program Ushikwapo Shikamana, they came together and decided to see the doctor for advice. I am very hopeful that they are going to succeed just like Kinga and Lulu."

(Kibet Simon 11/02/02)

"I am also grateful because I have been able to advise my fellow teachers and my students from the lessons I get from Ushikwapo Shikamana. I would advise the young men to desist from impregnating girls before marriage through irresponsible sex; and to the girls; they should keep off from men of bad behavior like Pangupangu. We must know that AIDS is real and we are the cure through responsible behaviors".

(Job Ambaka, Kisumu Ushikwapo Group, 20/06/02)

An impact evaluation study was carried out on the program' s fourth year. This was done by an independent research institution and evaluated the program based on the recognition of "markers", clinic exit data, letters, focus group discussions and in- depth interviews. Partner NGOs were also interviewed to determine if they found the program to be useful in their work- or to have increased demand for their services.

Despite the fact that it is challenging to peg down changes in society to a single program without bias a number of studies into the effectiveness of the program as a health intervention have found that the program has been effective in influencing some of these positive changes. Two studies will be highlighted in an effort to demonstrate the effectiveness of our intervention.

First is a study that was carried out in family planning clinics around the country with the objective to monitor listenership, reception and perception of the messages transmitted by the radio program. This was done through an in depth questionnaire that was designed and distributed to the Ministry of Health Maternal and Child Health (MCH) care facilities in five provinces; Coast, Rift Valley, Nyanza, Western and Eastern provinces.

The clinic questionnaire was specifically administered in the family planning units. In each province, four MCH facilities were targeted. The provinces were selected due to high listenership demonstrated by the number of listener letters received from these provinces. At the same time, the Monitoring Team selected these provinces to enable them capture listeners where it had not carried out focus group discussions. This was as a result of the cost of administering focus group discussions and the constraints in funding that did not make it possible for the Monitoring Team to travel into all the provinces.

The Monitoring Team in conjunction with National Nurses Association (NNAK) in cooperation with the Ministry of Health administered the clinic questionnaire. The National Nurses Association is the professional body of nurses in Kenya and has branches to the lowest health facility. The nurses most of who are members of NNAK are the health providers at maternal and health facilities. The nurses were therefore best placed to administer the clinic questionnaire. The Monitoring Team hoped to get better results by using the NNAK that has access to the nurse.

Of the total 1000 questionnaires sent out, 532 were returned to the Monitoring Team. The response was therefore slightly above 50%. The nurses were instructed to administer the questionnaire to the clients who attended the clinic for the first time. The nurse was asked to read the questions and not provide the answers and as the client answered, the nurse would tick a response as provided by the questionnaire.

Results from this study show that listeners continue to receive from Ushikwapo Shikamana Radio Programme a wealth of information on important issues that affect their health and well- being. The findings from the survey reveal that the listeners were in actual fact learning from the radio program. It is true that the radio series continues to be educative and beneficial to the target audience as they learn useful information. As information is power, we can conclude that the program continues to empower listeners with relevant day-to-day messages. Nyanza and Eastern Provinces returned most of the questionnaires while the response from the other provinces was below expectation. The reason for this was not forthcoming from the Chairpersons of the NNAK Branches responsible for the distribution of the questionnaires.

The questionnaire sought to gather information including the age of clients who attended the clinics; their marital status; what information the clients were seeking; what were the sources of the information sought and whether they had listened to *Ushikwapo Shikamana*. If they had, the client was then asked to highlight the information received from the radio program.

In all the health facilities over three-quarters of clients who attended the maternal and child health facility were married women and mostly of the ages 20 – 30 years. There were very few clients of the ages 15 – 20 and over 35 years. Most of the clients below 20 years were married. The clinic questionnaire also revealed that the young and unmarried women were not likely to attend the maternal and child health, as the number that attended the clinic of the ages 15-20 was negligible. The service these few young and unmarried women sought was mainly treatment for sexually transmitted infection. None indicated that they had come for family planning.

The clinic questionnaire sought to know the services/information the client sought from the health facility. The following table shows the response of the clients.

Table 1: Services the clients go for from MCH clinics

Province	Prenatal services	Family planning	STI Treatment	Check-up
Nyanza	68%	30%	2%	0
Eastern	70%	25%	5%	0
Western	60%	39%	1%	0
Coast	68%	29%	3%	0
Rift Valley	68%	30%	2%	0

Table 1 reveals that most of the clients who attended the health facility went for the prenatal services. The other need that was sought from the health facility was family planning. Apart from prenatal care and family planning, the women who attended the maternal and child health facilities were in need of STI treatment. No women indicated that they went to the clinic for normal check up. This is very important to note because, some illnesses such as cervical cancer are not possible to detect unless the women go for check ups. If women do not go for general check ups, then it is not possible to take preventive measures. That is why illnesses that could be prevented take toll on women because they are not detected early enough.

Discussion of family planning between couples

One of the most important issues in that determine the success or failure of family planning services is the openness/communication between couples on the number and the spacing of children a couple would like to have. The clinic questionnaire sought to know whether couples discussed or were making decisions together about family planning. The responses varied from province to province. In most provinces more than half of the couples (52%, Table 2.) reported to have discussed family planning. This is quite encouraging as this is one of the areas that those who participated in the formative research had expressed interest to have promoted in Ushikwapo Shikamana radio program.

Table 2: Couples who had discussed family planning in the last one month

	Nyanza	Eastern	Western	Coast	Rift valley	Total
Yes	100 (55%)	77 (42)	25 (45%)	23 (52%)	38 (56%)	263 (52%)
No	83 (45%)	94 (51%)	30 (55%)	17 (58)	29 (43%)	250 (48%)

Information on table 2 is very encouraging. If couples are discussing family planning, then total fertility rate will decline. This will contribute to positive development.

On the most important source of information clients came to know where to seek for services needed, the following were highlighted, friends and family, the next source the clinic and the last in important was the radio.

Table 3: The sources of information of where to seek services

Nyanza	Friend and family (32%)	Clinic (28%)	Radio (8%)
Eastern	Clinic (51%)	Friends and family (35%)	Radio (22%)
Western	Clinics (81%)	Friends and family (38%)	Radio (31%)
Coast	Friends and family (90%)	Clinic (31%)	Radio (13%)
Rift Valley	Friends and family (55%)	Clinic (40%)	Radio (12%)

From table 3, it is interesting to note that the clients who attended the maternal and child health clinics obtained information from either friends or clinics. The radio as a source of information came third in all provinces. This reflects the reality on the ground. Relative and friends influence most women while making such important decisions in life. The clinic is another credible source of information women may trust. It is unlikely that women will make decisions such as family planning from listening to the radio alone. The radio acts as a reinforcement of information already received from friends and clinics. Therefore, inter-personal communication seems to be a very important way of passing on crucial information.

What are the most important messages that the clients learnt from listening to *Ushikwapo Shikamana* radio series? The nurse administering the questionnaire was instructed not to read out the itemized messages but to let the participants call out what they had learnt. The following is the list of what the clients mentioned and listed in the order of what was mentioned most of the times and the number of times mentioned converted to percentages:

√ Family planning – 62%
√ HIV/AIDS- 57%
√ Communication between couples – 53%
√ Value of girls/women – 52%
√ Drugs and alcohol abuse – 52%
√ Issues of mother's heath- 47%

√ Issues of child's health – 45%

√ Economic issues – 43%

Below we review some letters that show the process of para-social interaction, namely "illusion of face to face relationship" that develop between a character and the audience. This suggests that Ushikwapo Shikamana is creating change in the minds of audience members.

Ushikwapo Shikamana being a prosocial media programs seeks to create directed and specified social change. Such programs aim to enhance self-efficacy and can foster desired behaviors. Studies on self-efficacy and programs that seek self-efficacy employ Bandura's social cognitive theory as an explanatory model. Bandura's self-efficacy theory (1992, 1995) argues that individuals will act in accordance with their perceived abilities to achieve what they desire.

In recent years, Bandura expanded the scope of self-efficacy functioning to include a self-reflective (1995, 1997) capability that regulates individual's motivations, thought processes and emotional states, as well as behavioural modifications. The self-reflective capability involves self-regulatory skills that include planning, organizing, regulating one's motivation, and applying metacognitive skills to evaluate the adequacy of one's knowledge and strategies.

Self-efficacy is both a belief and behavioural experience. When individuals wish to attain a goal, they point out their beliefs in their personal capabilities greatly determine the goal-setting and actuation processes. Efficacy is more like actuation.

Listeners' letters: Parasocial interaction and dimensions of self-efficacy

As indicated a radio program's capability to induce self-reflection amongst listeners enabling them to achieve self-efficacy in their lives is very much intertwined with the notion of parasocial interaction. It is through parasocial interaction that listeners appreciate the underlying values and challenges that a character faces. Parasocial interaction has also been used in the analysis of program effects in India (*Tinka Tinka Sukh*) and Tanzania (*Twende na Wakati*).

In *Ushikwapo Shikamana*, five types of parasocial interaction that demonstrate dimensions of self-efficacy were identified. However we will highlight three of these dimensions in this report.

Cognitively oriented para social interaction

Cognitively oriented parasocial interaction is the degree to which audience members pay particular attention to the characters in a media message and think about its educational content after their exposure (Papa et al., 1998; Sood & Rogers, 1996; Singhal & Rogers 1996: 172). A cognitive interaction therefore is an intellectual process, involving mainly the mind. In the case of the sample letters analyzed, cognitive interaction was the most dominant, demonstrating that the listeners grasped the educational issues infused into the radio drama.

In the study, of Ushikwapo Shikamana listener's letters by Kakai Karani (2002) at least 52 per cent of the letters exhibited cognitive awareness. As an aspect of self-efficacy, reflecting on the educational themes can help listeners recognize they have behavioural choices. (Singhal & Rogers 1999). Whereas we propose that cognitively oriented parasocial interaction is basic to self-efficacy in that behaviour change presupposes wholesome information, we are conscious 'that there is little evidence to date, however, that cognitively oriented interaction within a parasocial context can initiate a process of social change'. (Singhal & Rogers 1999: 173).

Here below we provide a translation (from Kiswahili) of an example of a co-written listeners' letter who demonstrate a clear knowledge (cognitive) of the educational issues. We have as much as possible preserved the original structure of the letter in our translation:

> Thank you for the programme 'Ushikwapo Shikamana'. It has taught us very much in many ways about the realities of current life. We say thank you very much and, if possible, we ask for an extension of the time of the programme.
>
> My views
>
> 1.   We congratulate Mwalimu Tatu and her fiancé Jaka for their decision to delay getting a baby.

2. We urge Chezi's husband to discard old customs and traditions because they can make him to lose his life. In addition, we urge him to construct a pit latrine.

3. We urge Mabuche to stop using drugs.

4. Shindo should stop dealing in hard drugs.

5. Inspector should stop receiving bribes and do his work with commitment. The way we see it, he is about to lose his job.

Yours faithfully,
Jaridah Machila and Ruth Wakto
Mwandago Secondary School
Po Box 161
Mwatate

Clearly, the notion of parasocial interaction is evident. The writers identify the educational issues involved and have been prompted to either offer advice or congratulate positive characters. The interaction helps to reinforce the listeners' sense of efficacy helping to enhance positive traits in their character.

Affectively oriented parasocial interaction

The emotional identification between members of the audience and media characters is a critical one in engendering feelings of self-efficacy. Affectively oriented parasocial interaction is the degree to which audience members identify with a particular media character. (Singhal & Rogers 1999). This bonding and identification influences the possibility of change. In the study, about 38 percent of letter writers exhibited affective interaction.

A range of letters demonstrated feelings of disgust, disapproval for bad behaviour, approval and recognition for prosocial behaviour. In the letter cited above, we can argue that both cognitive and affective interactions are mutually reinforcing.

Behaviorally oriented parasocial interaction

This dimension of parasocial interaction has been defined as the degree to which individuals overtly react to media characters. (Papa et al 2000). The reactions can facilitate change in the listener's own behaviour or motivate them to take specific action. Consider the following letter:

> To the Ushikwapo Programme
>
> I like other regular fans of the programme, listen to the programme every Saturday for the omnibus edition.
>
> If the truth be told, this programme has not only entertained me but it has also educated me and given me tips on how to write drama. I need your help so that I can write my play which will contribute to the development of Kiswahili. I also thank Mr. Ken Walibora for his book 'Siku Njema'. His book is an important contribution and has enriched my own life...
>
> Thank you
>
> Hellen Mabonga
> Sitatunga Primary School
> PO Box 3401
> Kitale

This particular letter is interesting for various reasons. The radio drama seems to trigger efficacy beyond the immediate objectives of the programme. First, the programme has inspired specific behavioural efficacy - the capacity to write and appreciate art and drama in particular. The listener's interest in writing and becoming an influential author is given specific force through the literary quality of the programme. For this particular listener, the programme is an opportunity to celebrate the wider objectives of art and its capacity to fulfill and affirm our humanity. She connects with the programme by recognizing writers who are not directly connected with the programme such as Ken Walibora, a newscaster with the Nation Media Group and author of the novel *Siku Njema*.

Self-efficacy is made possible through a process of parasocial interaction between audience members and media characters. We also contend that letters can provide first hand knowledge about how a radio programme affected an audience's sense of efficacy. Letters, written in response to a radio program are a scarcely studied area and they provide a genuine testimonial of how a program affects audience individuals.

Sustainability

Start-up costs for entertainment education programs are typically high, and such programs take a relatively longer time to produce than do strictly entertainment programs, in part due to the time and costs of formative evaluation research. On the other hand, entertainment-education programs have been found to be very efficient in achieving low-cost behaviour change (Singhal & Rogers 1999: 20).

Sponsorship: Though is hard to come by, Ushikwapo Shikamana has previously attracted sponsorship from the corporate world. Unga Ltd. who came on board and contributed a total of Ksh. 3,014,986 (approx. $38,400) towards the program. We ran one-minute Unga advertisement spots alongside Ushikwapo Shikamana and placed Unga products in the story- line once a week. Unga paid for.

VAT Exemption: The program has also been successful in getting exemption from paying VAT on some of our activities by Treasury which makes it a bit cheaper to produce and air the program. These exemptions were equivalent to production costs and airtime costs for 57 programs. This reduced costs by about $30,000 for the program.

Comic Book: In December 2001, *Ushikwapo Shikamana* Comic Book 1 was released. 5,000 copies were printed. The book is in full color. The Ministry of Education (Guidance and Counselling) and the Ministry of Culture (Adult Education division) find the book to be useful for young people. In December 2002 *Ushikwapo Shikamana* Comic Book 2 was released.

In conclusion, the Kenyan experience with *Ushikwapo Shikamana* for the past five years has many times emphasized the importance of social change programming proving that entertainment-education is a viable strategy of bridging the needless dichotomy between entertainment and education. *Ushikwapo Shikamana* is a concrete example of how entertainment and education can find common ground. The experience of *Ushikwapo Shikamana* presents interesting lessons on the opportunities and challenges of combining entertainment with educational messages for specific development objectives. Specifically, entertainment radio can be used to educate both young and old on a variety of issues.

Furthermore, formative research and impact evaluation are crucial to the success of entertainment-education. A balance between artistic creativity and communication research is needed in producing effective entertainment-education programs. Clearly, entertainment-education programs offer tremendous economies of scale delivering messages to a target audience.

VI

Culture as a Friend

There are those who mistakenly believe that culture is a barrier to health interventions. A more positive and accommodative view of culture is one which sees it in terms of its strengths and capabilities. Viewed as such, culture becomes a resource for HIV/AIDS prevention, care, and social support system. It becomes an opportunity and a space within which to work in dealing with major political, economic, social and environmental issues. Culture can be immensely facilitative if engaged positively. The replication of family ties in many societies in HIV/AIDS campaigns can, for example, play a major role in the fight against stigma, orphan-care and treatment. The invocation of socio-cultural and spiritual practices could create greater family harmony. It may provide spaces for communication on sensitive issues related to sexuality. Culture is also the space where effective communication strategies could be located. The oral narratives, proverbs, riddles and songs have tremendous capacity to communicate in a socially accepted manner.

Interesting programming work is being undertaken in Africa with the underlying understanding that culture can be a close ally. In order to see how culture is being used, the Soap Summit brought in people who are working with it. They were asked to think through these ideas.

(The panelists were Mr. Marvin Hanke from the Story Workshop, Malawi, Ms. Maungo Mooki of CDC, Botswana; and Alakie Mboya of Get Connected, Kenya. This session was chaired by Sam Mbure of AFMF, Kenya).

Marvin Hanke started the session by presenting a paper on *Linking Traditional Culture to Social Change*. He began by saying that Malawi has a wealth of proverbs used in daily conversation; to help settle disputes, express advice and make sense of people's life experiences. In his view, many traditional stories based on proverbs are actually parables or humorous situation tales which dramatize common mistakes people make based on greed, jealous and ambition. The meaning of specific proverbs illustrates the Story Workshop's approach, which is to tackle barriers to behaviour change through using culture as raw material for story telling and modeling, rather than simply forcing messages onto unwilling people. The story workshop uses proverbs as a way of responding to critical health, economic and gender issues.

Trying to push people to accept new ways of thinking and acting is futile if it is not linked to something already familiar and trusted. *Story Workshop's* educational media approach revolves around linking the values and beliefs in Malawian oral traditions and culture to the messages in their soap operas. They draw on the wisdom of their communities. Marvin Hanke said:

"*Story Workshop* is an educational media NGO in Malawi, blending culture and traditions with development messages on HIV/AIDS, food security and human rights. Using our edu-tainment techniques, we create radio soap operas, radio magazine programmes and debates, action theatre, music jingles, comic books and a host of other activities," he emphasized.

The story workshop has three radio soap operas on the National radio at the moment and every soap starts with a proverb which is tied to the objectives of that episode.

"Our most popular radio show, *Zimachitika* ("Such is Life") - is listened to by more than half of the country." For the past four years Zimachitika has been voted the number one radio drama in the country in the yearly Entertainers Awards, and it also won the Commonwealth Award for Action on HIV/AIDS. This success is attributed to the unique way chosen to link culture with social change." These recognitions are manifestation of the reception that the strategy draws.

"Culture is often viewed by donors and development practitioners as a barrier to progress, and is often used to explain development failures. Experiences drawn from Story Workshop have shown that culture can also be used to break barriers to progress - for example, if women have to traditionally sit on the floor in the presence of men, some people protest that changing that is breaking their culture. But that simply isn't the case. We all know that culture is dynamic. We no longer make human sacrifices to the gods. Even though this was part of our culture in the past it is not our culture today."

Contraversially, Hanke argued that cognitive processing differs within people of different nationalities; a difference shaped by their environment. Without going into the sapir-whorf hypothesis in which language is seen to shape thought yet seemingly inspired by it, Hanke argued for an appreciation of local knowledge and information processing. An endorsement of a strong version of this hypothesis is of course dangerous, because it could be used to disempower people. Yet a softer version related to indigenous knowledge could be quite enriching. According to Hanke:

"One of the key failures of many behaviour change initiatives is that they assume that people think the same way. Western designed interventions assume that Africans, Latin Americans and Asians think the same way as Americans or Norwegians. If you tell a Malawian that they should get rid of mosquitoes to get rid of malaria, they will not agree that it is vital and start sleeping under a bed net immediately. This is because many Malawians believe that you get malaria from getting wet in the rain or eating sugarcane that is not ripe– after all the malaria season and the rainy season (which also happens to be the time sugarcane starts growing) coincide. Unless you make a connection between the water pools (breeding areas for mosquitoes) and the prevalence of mosquitoes during the rainy season, or the sugarcane story, your messages will make no sense to your target audience."

Story Workshop links new ideas with traditional, familiar ways of doing things and thinking about them. Culture, therefore, can be used as material for storytelling and modeling new ways for communities to survive and thrive.

They believe development messages need to fit the social context of a community and that the information which unfolds through the authentic conflict and resolution of drama is more likely to be adsorbed into the thoughts and actions of daily life. Through the problems and struggles of popular story characters, listeners experience familiar issues and challenges while learning new ways of coping with threats to community survival. The story workshop views culture as an ally.

The Story Workshop takes traditional characters and helps them to be pragmatic to today's needs and setting. One of the characters, an old woman (Gogo) uses her heritage of traditional stories and proverbs to link important cultural values to changing social and economic realities faced by her grandchildren. She likens consultation in modern democracies to consultations among people in her clan during funerals. She will argue in favour of family planning by explaining that in her time there was a lot of land and very few people to farm the land. Today, the opposite is true and that dictates that we plan our families.

The Story workshop has a Music Ensemble, which is an acapella and traditional rhythm group using a mix of hand-built and modern instruments, drums and choral voices. Every show has songs that blend traditional music and modern music to enforce the proverbs, parables, and messages for the story; in the process, adding to the entertainment itself.

In summary, they use culture as story resource and a catalyst for social change, and they believe that soap operas help change lives.

Maungo Mooki, made a presentation on *Barriers and Facilitators to Achieving Objectives to Health Situations.* She began by defining culture as values of a group as well as ideals and beliefs over a lifetime. Her organisation produces a drama, which focuses on behavior. The issues include positive prevention, voluntary counseling, prevention of HIV transmission from mother to child, and anti-retroviral therapy.

She then looked at culture as a barrier to achieving their objectives and pointed out that the first issue is positive prevention, which involves limiting alcohol intake, delayed marriages and pregnancies, and limiting partners. Barriers to this include arranged marriages, polygamy, condom stigma, unsafe breastfeeding practices, and alcohol taking on all occasions. Care begins at home and this home-based care (HBC) is done in unsafe conditions and those taking care end up being infected. VCT centres are already stigmatized because of HIV and the fact that the condition is associated with promiscuity.

And in looking at culture as a facilitator, the 'SOTHO' phenomenon where respect for others, particularly older people and people in authority becomes key. The extended family set up (UBUNTU) support structure and mechanism, as well as the 'KGOTLA' system of doing things together/consultative forums do facilitate.

Mooki gave some of the lessons learnt in the process: that it is important to use and incorporate culture in drama to make it appealing to local audiences. It is also important to use culture to make the drama realistic and relevant and acknowledge where culture can be an obstacle and try to incorporate it.

Alakie Mboya pointed out that culture can be classified into three categories namely artifacts, norms and behaviour. In order to create behavioral change, we must have concerted efforts. Language has to be understood in order to use the right language for the youth.

'Get connected' is a youth programme that she produces. This radio drama has been translated into small booklets. The programme has an editorial committee. The aspiration for the programme is that it can be translated into a television series.

Things to ponder about:

- Do producers involve young people in designing messages? How about in implementation?

- How do you avoid stereotyping communities? How do you ensure linguistic sensitivity?

A major challenge which culture presents to us is communication on sensitive sexual issues. These are discussions that are viewed as taboo. Within the context of HIV/AIDS greater communication channels between generations need to be opened.

VII

Interpersonal and Inter-generational Communication

One of the critical challenges facing contemporary Africa in the era of globalization is poor interpersonal and intergeneration communication. The youth look for icons from other parts of the world other than in their immediate environment. They are impatient with life and want quick solutions to their predicament. They are fighting with time which is slow in coming. On the other hand, older people are unimpressed by the influence of media; they think young people have lost direction. The era of liberation and openness brings with it opportunities and new dilemmas.

How is programming work being undertaken to address this issue?
(The panelists at this session were: Oby Obyerodhiambo of PATH, Kenya; Margaret Adaba of Communication for Change, Nigeria; Donna Sherard of Family Care International, Kenya and Mia Malan, Internews, UK. This session was chaired by Alakie Mboya).

Oby Obyerodhiambo made a presentation on *'Sorting out Babel' Making Interpersonal and Intergenerational Communication Work.'*

He began by pointing out that the biblical tower of Babel describes with great accuracy the current state of reproductive health communication in Africa, and probably the entire world. Individuals have difficulty communicating to the next person, their partners, friends and even enemies. Parents are unable to reach to their children and children are unable to communicate to their elders. Women are unable to talk to their brothers, partners, spouses, in-laws and entire communities. It is no wonder that the phrase, "You see what I am saying?!" has become a rather monotonous interjection in speech. Interpersonal and cross-generation communication has never been at such a point of crisis. In the urban areas this communication is made even worse by the centrality of television and other non-interpersonal communication tools.

This presentation attempted to analyze the obstacles to communication at the personal and the cross generation level and then suggest ways in which these can be overcome. He illustrated how the PATH Kenya designed *Kati Yetu* radio program has tried to increase the interpersonal and inter-generation communication within the Impact project sites in Mombasa (now expanding to Kilifi and Malindi), Nakuru and Western Province.

Oby said: "Inter-personal communication today faces several challenges. Since we are confining our scope to Africa in this discussion, we dare say that many of these challenges have a genesis in colonialism and the subsequent break up of the traditional structures of the societies. A word of caution on the outset is that some of the results of colonialism and westernization have indeed enhanced communication especially in terms of the expansion of mass media.

The first challenge to interpersonal communication faced today is the lack of the opportunity, the forum or the time to communicate. In the pre-colonial past individuals within a community were relatively closed in within their communal dwellings. They had unlimited access to each other over a greater part of their waking time. Their lives revolved round relatively common events in very tight geographical confines. Socialization processes in varied communities provided a forum where various age-sets (peers) communicated among themselves. Hence the opportunity to communicate, that today is a major challenge to interpersonal communication, was not a real problem then. Today, because of mass migrations, social disruptions like children going off to school early in the morning and returning late in the evening (or even going to work in coffee and tea plantations) has taken away both the time and forum for interpersonal communication at the family and community level.

Neither is the modern formal school system communication friendly. The most often heard reprimand in school is, 'Silence' or, 'Keep Quiet'. In some educational institutions conversation even outside of class is very restricted. The formal education system is a typical one-way information street that inculcates a culture of introspection as opposed to interpersonal communication. The burden of homework and assignments ensures that the child returns home and has to remain sullen as he or she grapples with the work alone. Those who are unfortunate to be among the myriad child laborers in Africa are too exhausted by the end of the day to communicate to anybody. The communal sharing of meals and sleeping-mat that provided the opportunity for the tales of yore is at best lost.

On a larger scale, the urbanization of Africa has created a new multi-ethnic and multi-cultural urban community that share almost nothing. In the slums, life is too tough to allow the opportunity for spontaneous interpersonal communication while in the more affluent dwellings the high walls and electrified fences ensure that every family unit is locked within their own little world. Not only are the opportunities for communication lost but common interest and shared concerns do not exist. There is hardly a shared perspective on reproductive health issues.

At another level, culture and socialization creates yet another barrier to interpersonal communication. First, there is the loss of the specialist culture-bound language that was used to communicate about issues relating to sex and sexuality. Secondly, social etiquette makes it difficult in many communities for the free discussion of matters of sex and sexuality. Sex and sexuality were discussed in very specific settings and in very specific terms. Once these special forums that facilitated this communication are lost a gap results. The sex-talk is carried on in a social vacuum and this leads to stigmatization and discomfort.

Furthermore, the socialization results in a situation where future interpersonal communication between sexual partners is not possible. Sex is a taboo subject. Sexually transmitted infections including HIV is stigmatized. This attitude is carried right through into marriage and spouses cannot discuss their sexual issues and reproductive health matters. So not only are audience and opportunity to communicate reproductive health issues lost, but the language to communicate it too.

Religion, and especially Christianity and Islam have, in Africa, created yet another barrier to communication on reproductive health issues. The attitude towards sex and sexuality in these religions has rendered it a taboo subject. The more spiritual one becomes in these the less they are allowed to talk about sex, let alone engage in it. Religion elevated sex and sexuality from a physical to a spiritual dimension.

Talking about sexuality became a spiritual aberration and was discouraged.

Turning to the intergenerational communication, the biggest obstacle is the moralistic-judgmental attitude held by the older generation which is countered by the dismissive and 'you know nothing' attitude of the youth. The generational conflict that arises renders inter-generation communication all but impossible. The elders engage in moral bludgeoning of the younger generation and the holier than thou attitude creates an environment that is not conducive to communication.

Language, or rather the lack of it, is another challenge to intergenerational communication. Language operates here at two levels; there is the fact that many young people do not speak the language that their grandparents or parents speak well enough to allow communication, especially the subtlety that communicating reproductive health issues calls for. Secondly, is the register used by the youth. The older generation is unable to communicate to the youth in their youthful hip-hop lingo. This is compounded by the 'youth register' that seems to communicate about sex and sexuality in explicit terms. In Kenya, for example, the sheng slang cuts off older people from the world of the youth.

Generally the African culture also creates a barrier between the youth and the older generation. There are issues that cannot be discussed between a father and daughter, or mother and son. In the pre-colonial past the communal living provided for a forum in which somebody else filled that communication gap. Today, and the case of single parents is even worse, there is a tendency to cling on to the cultural taboos that restricted the discussion on sexuality, whereas the social support systems that filled that gap are no longer present.

The forum for intergeneration communication has shrunk over time. The forums that existed in the past where the elders came together with the youth are no longer viable with urbanization and nuclearization of the families."

Oby Obyerodhiambo argued that their existed spaces for intergenerational communication now significantly eroded by urbanization, technologization and globalization. More creative ways of facilitating communication within the contemporary world would need to be sought. He posed a question and then answered it:

"Since it is not possible to turn the clock back to the pristine times, how can we enhance interpersonal and intergeneration communication especially on reproductive health matters?

Radio has emerged as the answer to the problem of forum and opportunity. This is what makes the radio the most potent tool to bridge this gap. The all pervasive nature of the radio and its relative affordability renders it a viable tool to reach a large cross section of the population. Through radio programming it is possible to de-stigmatize sex, sexuality and STIs. Radio allows us the benefit of 'planting' issues of RH within communities by creating some cognitive dissonance that will lead to discussion. Through radio, taboo topics and issues can be seeded into the community and elevated to issues for discussion. For example, the condom has become a common topic for discussion because the radio was able to plant it as an issue within communities. The process of setting up communal dilemmas forces the communities to communicate among themselves. The radio assists this process by offering them information of the same subject.

The radio, and here the radio soap becomes very useful, is able to objectify the reality and thereby allow for discussions on the fictional plane of issues that cultural and religious taboo make difficult to confront. The fictional world created by the soaps allows for the critical examination of sex and sexuality."

Oby then used *Maisha ya Nuru* a segment of the *Kati Yetu* Radio program to illustrate.

Kati Yetu is divided into two major segments: the radio soap opera – *Maisha ya Nuru* and the Radio magazine section that has interviews, discussions, quizzes, vox-pop and health news. The radio program is a complimentary component of the peer-education intervention. There are listening groups – radio groups- in the project areas that meet every week to listen to the program. They are also sent tapes of the program every week so that they can review the program and use it in their discussions. There is a Discussion Guide that the implementer of the Program (PATH-Kenya) prepares to allow a richer discussion among the radio groups. The questions from the group discussions are fed back to the program.

The radio groups are found within the target population of sex workers, low income community women and men and women in the work site. By creating these radio groups an opportunity for interpersonal discussion is created.

The Radio soap, *Maisha ya Nuru* has an interesting dynamic in that it is really the story of a young woman Nuru, who goes through life confronted by the daily issues of relationships. As she relates to different segments of her community, issues of interpersonal and intergenerational communication are played out. She relates to her peers, her parents, and others. Through this radio soap PATH has been able to re-create a modern communication forum; a family unit living within a society. Within this community there are relationship issues that they need to confront and discuss. They have been able to plant controversial issues and have the characters discuss them. For example the Radio soap *Maisha ya Nuru* has allowed them to have an African man discuss sexuality with his 'daughter', which is a taboo. The questions that this raises in the community of listeners lead to a debate on the viability of such discussions in real life.

The radio program also deals with issues that emerge from the youth targeted community theatre outreaches. The youth who listen to the radio soap and have identified with the main character, Nuru, are able to feed into the questions that the radio magazine section deals with. Through the re-enactment of various segments of Nuru in the Magnet theatre outreaches the youth specific issues are discussed in a forum that brings together a diverse age group. A typical theater outreach will have the target audience; youth between the ages of 10-25 as well as children and adults. All these groups will also be keen listeners of the radio program. There is a communicative loop that all these groups fit into.

Finally as part of the entire intervention there is the Nuru Comic book. The comic book has been developed up to volume three and is targeted at youth in and out of school. The radio soap opera and the comic book are slowly working towards merging since they started off at different trajectories. However the main character is the same and the challenges she faces are similar.

In Conclusion, Oby posited that in order to enhance interpersonal and intergenerational communication there is need to re-create forums in which individuals and communities can come together to interact. Radio seems to play a significant role here, especially the more interactive and participatory radio program. Secondly, there is need to create an environment that allows for the discussion of sensitive matters. The taboo subjects, the cultural 'no-go' areas, will need to be mediated by the objectification of reality through the fictional soaps. Once the issues are planted in the community they become common discussion topics and the stigma value dies out. To do this the radio must be provocative and controversial if it is to create adequate cognitive dissonance. The communal dilemmas that the radio generates will force communication on the issues. Finally, the radio forum will be able to provide a source of correct and reliable information to counter the myths and misconceptions and the promiscuous sources of information."

The opening up of space for interpersonal and intergenerational communication is also being undertaken in Eritrea through the Romadi radio soap opera. Romadi opens up opportunities for a magazine segment – discussion, news, proverb, music – and a comic strip in the local daily. The project design also includes listening clubs. Drawing on experiences with the Maisha ya Nuru project, the African Youth Alliance project in Tanzania especially the Mambo Bomba radio youth variety show, and Ushikwapo Shikamana, Romadi is likely to have an impact in Eritrea.

In order to understand how Nigeria is dealing with these issues, we invited Adaba to the panel.

Margaret Adaba, made a presentation on *Changing Images of Africa: Voices of Urban Youth*. She began by pointing out that some time back, a caption of one issue of the *Economist* magazine's cover page was "*Africa, the Hopeless Continent*", picturing an African revolutionary in his mid-twenties, toting a gun inside the map of Africa. A few months later, the same news magazine had a close up of a young black child on the front cover with the words 'poverty, disease and debt' superimposed over it. Another print advert for the BBC showed a teenage African boy with a red bandana and blood soiled, torn clothes pointing a bazooka gun in the sky with the caption, " *One international decision-maker you won't find in the boardroom*". On CNN, a Sierra Leone journalist presented a harrowing account of the years he spent covering the war – the most devastating part of the film was the in-depth look at child soldiers, and how they terrorize the entire civilian population. These are the daily images we see of Africa and African youth in the international press.

Adaba went on to say:

"In Nigeria, youth have for the most part been cast in an equally combative and violent role as they appear to be at the forefront of most ethnic and religious conflict. In the Niger Delta, the Ijaw youth resistance has brought the region to its knees with guerrilla warfare. During ethnic clashes in many parts of the country, it is the youth who seem to spearhead the rioting, killing, looting and maiming. If it is not outright fighting that is being reported on, then young people have grabbed center stage through stories of cults and inter-gang warfare on university campuses across the nation.

Surely these stereotypes of youth in Nigeria and Africa present a very skewed image of the average young person on the continent. Is it that the international and African press are unaware of more realistic and complex stories? Or that they don't have access to the complete life worlds of African youth?

Taken separately, these images are not untrue. Neither are the images of rock throwing in Ramala or of student shootings in Colorado in and of themselves, untrue. None of them are, however, representative of day to day life in Nigeria or in Palestine or in the United States. It is, in short, their woeful incompleteness that creates a falsehood. On the one hand they provide only a very narrow glimpse of cultures that are complex, dynamic, multidimensional. These images of Africa, for example, find the sensational and the exotic. They are the easy stories because their drama is intense, raw, and in-your-face. They do not require the crafting of an event with all the dull parts of every day life taken out. There is a problem, however, when it is only these stories that get told and not those that can be found with an investigating and inquiring search. When it is only this that others see of us, then it is only this that they know of us. When it is only this that we see of ourselves, then we come to believe that this is who we are.

We need a wider view, and we also need a deeper view. These images of violence, of the exotic and the strange are really just that –

images. They are not the whole story, or even the real story. When the youth of the Niger Delta or in Palestine or in Colorado engage in violence it is dramatic, but it is not the story. Rather, the violence is a vehicle for sending a message; it is a symptom, a clue. The real story lies somewhere in the day to day realities of every day people as they live and make sense of their lives.

How do we address the falsehood created by both a breadth and depth of incompleteness perpetrated by broadcasting about Africa? If these images of poverty, disease and violence as well as of the exotic are not the real stories of Africa, then what are? And how do we find them? And why is it important that we do?"

Adaba called for a critical reconsideration of how Africa is presented in the world. A significant part of this realignment would have to be undertaken by creative writers and artists from Africa. She illustrated these efforts with her own experience in developing *Ready or Not*, a 52 episode radio drama series supported by the Rockefeller and Ford Foundation. During the past two years the series has been broadcast on thirty-seven radio stations throughout Nigeria, with both English and Hausa versions, and was presented in the United States at the MOJA Festival of African-American and Caribbean art.

The radio drama grew from an interest in the convergence of Nigeria's urban youth, development issues and social conflict in an emerging democracy. A central theme of the drama was finding the authentic voice of Nigerian youth and giving them a chance to express themselves on the air. The producers of *Ready or Not* sought to get at the real stories, the day to day lived realities of those who would be responsible for Nigeria's tomorrow. The project team found these stories through intensive grass roots research with youth (aged 13-29 years of age) throughout Nigeria and developed them into the radio drama by engaging youth throughout the production process.

Their voices tell stories which are real stories with hope and optimism that things will get better, reflecting young people's creativity, "joie de vivre", and bubbly enthusiasm for reaching new horizons, and breaking through stifling norms. They also tell stories of abuse, of institutionalised corruption, of adolescent vice within a wider, more realistic context.

These stories emerged and were developed using a formative media research design process which works from the bottom-up (or the inside-out) to find and develop program content. These are the real stories of Nigeria's urban youth and this is how they were found. The radio listeners tell us why it is important to find and broadcast these stories.

In terms of real stories, there is no question that the lives of urban youth in Nigeria are touched by AIDS, ethnic violence, and poverty. Yet the picture of devastation, senseless sacrifice, and hopeless condemnation, that the dominance of these images in world broadcasting implies, is not the whole of their world. When youth were invited to speak for themselves, they described a richer, deeper, and much more complex picture. The authenticity of their hopes and their fears, of their conflicts and their dreams of a better tomorrow is captured instead in the stories created by an ensemble of characters like themselves in the infotainment drama *Ready or Not*.

T.J. at twenty-three is a student, working part time as a DJ, while Fortune at twenty-five, having been expelled from school, is idle and non-productive. He smokes, drinks, gambles and lies. His younger sister Cynthia, though stuck in the gap between secondary school and university, is ambitious, and while street-wise, tries to stay on the straight and narrow until she can begin her studies in law. Other youths include Prince who although disabled, will not let his lack of working legs keep him from getting ahead, and Lucky, who has the name but not the luck. He is a street boy that missed a lot of opportunities and now drifts, mixing dubious cons. Simply Sofie, at age 22, is saucy, snobbish, smart and sensuous, and because of her experience, the one girls run to when they are in trouble. Young Austin, at 18, is a bit nerdy, working part time as a computer analyst and as an intern as he awaits the end of a strike so that he can go back to school. There is also a proud journalist in this mix of youth, Henry, whose column often gets him and others in trouble.

These youths come together regularly at the Hope Rising Recreational Center, where they find T.J.'s joint "MasterVibes" an attractive meeting place. Hope Rising Recreational Center also brings the world of adults into their lives, some helpful, some annoying. Joy Seka owns the center, and works tirelessly to ensure that the youth get the most out of it. Her strength and political aspirations often put her in conflict with another adult, Barrister Williams, the Chairperson of the local government. Sarge is Hope Rising's security officer, and as a retired army officer, never tires of recalling tales. Kaltume at 30 provides a motherly presence as the counselor that youth know they can trust, and Captain provides leadership as the coach of the disabled football team and frequent youth advocate.

For a glimpse at what are the real struggles urban youth in Nigeria face one need only listen to the experiences that they share when they are given a chance to speak and be heard in focus group discussions. Young men and young women are forced to put up with an under funded school system, strikes, and exam malpractice in their attempt to get an education. Youth suffer from the childhood lost in the dangers inherent in exposing children to street trading in an effort to combat poverty. Those young women who are victims of sexual abuse and rape, rarely find justice. The society equally rejects young women when prostitution is the only option they see for survival. Early childhood marriage has far-reaching effects on the health, social and psychological well being of girls who are not allowed to make their own choices. Youths get trapped in peer pressure and its extreme, cultism, and they find themselves tempted by the promise of drugs as a way out of pain. Youths are faced with the demands of traditional African values and the influence of Western cultures. The young face a lot of difficulties in seeking gainful employment, and girls are doubly affected by discrimination. Youth are disappointed when their expectations of the media to be fair and responsible are dashed. Youth care about the environment and they are frustrated with the short term thinking of their elders. These experiences are the stories of *Ready Or Not*.

While one could argue what is more positive in these stories, it is important to note that they are realistic, complex and multi-layered, set against a backdrop of dynamic, enthusiastic and inspiring characters. There is also a compelling sense of hope and optimism. When youth speak they do not express a sense of despair, of helplessness, or of devastation that dominant images in world broadcasting imply. While realistic, rather than idealistic, they are positive about the possibilities of their future in Nigeria.

The characters and the stories of *Ready or Not* are as complex, as contradictory, and as conflicting as the youth that they are about. They are the stories that lie beneath the images of violence and irresponsibility, and they believe the easy stereotypes. One has to look a little harder to find these dramas. But they are there, in the everyday lives of the youth of Nigeria.

With regards to program design and developing the content of 'real life' drama, the first stage of the formative research revealed that an underlying problem of urban conflict and violence found to be spearheaded by youth was the lack of opportunity that youth felt for their voices to be heard and taken seriously. The most important factor underlying this problem was their lack of access to the mainstream discourse. Thus, while Nigeria was feeling the fresh air of a new democratic revival, youth perceived that there was not a place at the table for their inputs. Accordingly, the design challenge of *Ready or Not* was defined as one of facilitating the access of youth's perspective to the discursive space of Nigeria's new future.

The second stage of the formative research addressed issues of program design. There was a need to close the gap between the life worlds or social realities of professional media designers and the life worlds of urban youth as well as their understandings of development issues. This was accomplished through a qualitative research design involving a youth forum, focus groups, and youth reporters. The purpose of this research was to gain entry to the world of meanings held by Nigeria's youth that could be captured in the creation of characters, settings, plots and themes of the 52 episode radio drama. Meanings about youth were also sought from groups of working class adults.

The primary objective of the qualitative research was, in short, to find the voice of youth, to find their stories. Projective exercises captured even richer layers of meanings relevant to the life world experiences of Nigeria's youth. The results of one of the projective exercises in which youths were asked to design their own complimentary card revealed a very independent, entrepreneurial streak – most saw themselves as executive or managing directors, chief consultants of their own organizations and business ventures.

With another exercise, young people were asked to imagine Nigeria as a car, and then to identify who or what would be its various parts. The youth identified the media as positive and pivotal. They characterized the media as Nigeria's headlights, "forward looking, with foresight, taking the long view, " as its shock absorbers, "absorbing the bumps," as Nigeria's engine, "converting the energy, spreading enthusiasm, and whirling ideas," and as the steering wheel, "keeping Nigeria going in the right direction." Nigeria's youth put a lot of faith and trust in the media. Youth also characterized themselves as Nigeria's headlights, and, along with human rights groups, NGO's and policy makers as Nigeria's petrol, "supplying energy, ideas and enthusiasm." But, they also saw themselves, along with the flag and government officials, as the car logo, "out in front, polished, looking good but not contributing much."

This rich layer of meanings provided an entree to the ambiguities and contradictions that life worlds naturally hold. Some traditional values were good, for example, while others were oppressive. They provide insights into the complexity of behavior and motivation as well as the conditionality of opinions and attitudes that begin to tell the "real" stories of a culture's life world.

As concerns the production design, the formative research revealed both the lifestyle preferences of youth and their media preferences, influencing the form and style of *Ready or Not*. Because the research revealed that young people all over Nigeria like to listen to music in their free time, or listen to radio and television dramas, the project team decided to produce a radio drama with a strong focus on music. Also the youths in most parts of northern Nigeria expressed their almost exclusive preference for local language dramas. Therefore the production team decided to reallocate production funds so that a Hausa version of the programme could be produced.

Another contribution to the finding of "real" stories was the empowerment of youth themselves. Youth were trained as special assignment reporters and sent out to interview youth about such things as life styles, media preferences, and heroes. They were also trained to become the scriptwriters for the series. They learned not only how to write compelling drama, but to do it from the perspective of the research findings. In addition, youth were recruited to produce the title song for the series as well as the music video, and young people were cast as the actors in both the English and the Hausa versions of the series, after receiving acting and speech classes from the project's veteran director.

Ready or Not went on air in April 2000, and by September, twenty stations nationwide were airing the English series and eleven stations were airing the Hausa series. Reactions from broadcasters was overwhelmingly positive, with each station agreeing to air the program during weekend prime time slots with at least one repeat during each week.

Preliminary reactions from young people and adults' were recorded during six focus group discussions held in key locations (a secondary school, a university campus, an urban youth centre and an urban, high-density, low income neighborhood) during October 2000, seven months after the series was launched. The respondents listened to three sample programs dealing with peer pressure, rape and conflict resolution, and commented that the programs were positive because they portrayed true-life situations and experiences, reflected valuable lessons of life, and were capable of inducing positive change in society. During some of the episodes, the emotions evoked among the youth were quite intense, reflecting an inner resolve to deal with the issues raised. Eighty-eight percent of respondents felt the stories were real and true to life, ninety one percent felt the messages were very clear and 92% felt the lessons in the drama were important for youth. Ninety-four percent of respondents felt the stories were entertaining and interesting and 85% agreed they would recommend the series to their family and friends and would listen to more episodes.

It is important that we find and tell the 'real' stories. As the audience reactions show, it is fundamentally important that a culture or a people or a person have the opportunity to define its reality. Images of African youth bear little resemblance to the life worlds of the majority of Africans, yet they are defining the reality that is Africa, not only for the rest of the world, but for Africans as well," Adaba concluded.

One of the ways of getting the real stories, that Adaba is encouraging us to go for, is to consciously create spaces for the voices of the youth. They ought to be involved right from the beginning of the intervention and allowed to articulate their interpretation of the world. Through a process of nurturing and mentoring, the youth can help realign the world.

We also wanted to learn about the development of materials related to youth and sexuality.

Donna Sherard made a presentation on *Health Education Materials for African Adolescents*. She said that in 1997, Family Care International (FCI) set out to develop a set of materials on sexuality and reproductive health for adolescents in English-speaking Africa to help ensure that they have the information and skills they need to make healthy and responsible choices about sexual activity. After a two-year development process, the materials — *Stepping Out*, a video series with an accompanying discussion guide, and *You, Your Life, Your Dreams*, an information handbook for adolescents — were produced in late 1999 and early 2000.

She went on to elaborate:

"Since producing the materials, FCI has distributed approximately 3,800 copies of *Stepping Out* and 6,500 copies of *You, Your Life, Your Dreams*. As part of the distribution efforts, a series of orientation and training workshops were held to introduce the materials to local partners in Ghana, Kenya and Uganda and help them integrate the set into their planned and ongoing work with adolescents. In follow-up to these activities, FCI conducted an evaluation of the materials to solicit feedback on the materials from adolescents and those working with youth. The evaluation focused on the feedback received from users who completed and returned written questionnaires distributed with each copy of the materials, as well as in-depth and group interviews with users and members of the materials' target audiences.

Evaluation forms, which were enclosed in each copy of *You, Your Life, Your Dreams* and *Stepping Out*, were one of the main vehicles for soliciting feedback from users of the materials. The evaluation forms included a range of questions aimed at gathering both quantitative and qualitative feedback on each resource, along with suggestions for improvement in case subsequent editions are produced.

Because experience in the evaluation and survey methodology has shown that relatively few people complete and return surveys, the evaluation forms included a special offer of additional copies of the materials, free of charge, for those who returned the completed evaluation questionnaires. In addition, the project partners sent out E-mail and letter reminders in early 2001 to those who had received copies of the materials, requesting recipients to take a few moments to complete and return the evaluation questionnaires.

Despite the above efforts, very few evaluation forms were returned; the response rate for each of the two materials was less than 1%. All but one of the completed evaluation questionnaires were returned by recipients in Africa, with most of the respondents being from Ghana and Uganda. Other respondents were from Kenya, Nigeria, South Africa and Tanzania. Feedback on each resource is summarized below:

A. You, Your Life, Your Dreams

The majority of the respondents were peer educators and youth counselors. However, a few teachers and health workers also returned the evaluation questionnaires, along with two adolescents—one from Ghana and another from South Africa. Most of the respondents reported that they were using the book as a reference for counseling young people or leading educational programs with young people, however many respondents indicated that they were also using it as the basis for developing additional health education materials.

Overall, respondents rated the book highly—4.3 on a scale of 1 to 5—and gave positive appraisals of the book's relevance (4.7) and cultural appropriateness (4.2). Respondents also indicated that they found the book enjoyable to read (4.6) and that the level of language was easy for adolescents to understand (4.4). The adolescent respondents consistently gave the book higher ratings than did non-adolescents; adolescents gave the book an overall rating of 5, compared with non-adolescents, who rated the book 4.2.

Almost no chapters were cited as "least useful", almost every chapter was cited by a respondent as "most useful", especially the chapters on relationships, sexuality, sexual health, pregnancy, emotional health, unwanted sex, planning for the future and hygiene and nutrition. One of the adolescent respondents noted that all chapters are "equally and vitally relevant and useful." However, it was suggested that additional information on getting along with parents and parental relationships be added to the book.

Respondents also reported that none of the chapters were culturally inappropriate, with one user writing: "I find the way the chapters were presented as culturally sensitive" and another commenting: "we live in a changing world which is very challenging—therefore all of the chapters are quite appropriate."

Interestingly, while a few adult respondents expressed some concern that the book might be too large, dense or difficult for young people to understand (e.g. "The volume of the book is too huge that the adolescent may get discouraged but if possible user more cartoons and photographs"), adolescent respondents gave the highest possible rating (5) to the book's size, language level, and appeal/accessibility (i.e. whether the book was enjoyable to read). In their written feedback, adolescents were also positive about the book, noting: "The size, layout, binding are all excellent...." and "Thank you 1,000 times to all the people who contributed to making these resources so appropriate, culturally sensitive, and inspiring."

The book's glossary was among the most highly rated aspects of the book, rated 5 by all respondents. As one adolescent commented: "The glossary is excellent because of the number of words it defines and we understand. You, Your Life, Your Dreams has helped me a lot." Other respondents commented: "The glossary was very necessary since some words may be obvious to a group of adolescents while others may not" and "the definitions [are] well understood. Good work".

The chapter summaries and "Did you know...boxes" (text boxes containing factual information) were also highly rated, particularly by adolescents, who rated each of these features 5, whereas adult respondents rated the chapter summaries and text boxes 4.9 and 4.6, respectively. As one respondent noted: "The summary boxes are quite useful as someone who may not have grasped the lengthy chapter may do so in the summary. Also someone who is in a hurry may need the summary box and get enough ideas." Another respondent wrote of the text boxes: "This part of the book taught me how I should advise the youth and was very easy to understand. Keep it up. It also helps you to make a decision."

Two aspects of the book that were rated more highly by adults than by adolescents were the illustrations/cartoons and the quotes from young people about their experiences and perspectives on adolescence. Adolescent respondents gave the illustrations and quotes slightly lower ratings (4 and 3, respectively), than did adult respondents (4.1 and 4.2, respectively). Nonetheless, respondents indicated that the illustrations and quotes were well linked to the text, and most reported that the book contained the right number of quotes and illustrations. Additionally, written feedback about the illustrations and quotes was very positive:

- "The illustrations and the cartoons are a great attraction for the adolescents. Well done."
- "Some of the adolescents' quotes [are] some of the things as the writer put up, [and] the illustrations hit on the top of the nail, keep it up!"
- "The book is good. All illustrations and linkages are well designed. We are most grateful."

Respondents also offered a few suggestions for improving the illustrations, such as coloring the illustrations to make them more appealing and interesting to adolescents (noted by two adult respondents); and adding additional illustrations.

Other general comments and suggestions about the book included:

- "The book should have been divided into parts to make it easier for the adolescents to read. Most of the adolescents may not have time to go through this book because of the size."
- "This book is very useful to me, my family, and our associates. We are in a farming village and cleanliness and exercise is very essential. This book has taught us a lot and we look forward to more."

B. *Stepping Out* (video & discussion guide)

Respondents were representatives of government institutions (e.g. health facilities) and local non-governmental organizations from Uganda and Tanzania, who reported that they had used the series in a variety of ways, including: using the entire series in the course of six separate sessions; conducting an intensive one-day session going through each of the video modules and follow-up discussion sessions; and playing the video modules on a continuous basis, without follow-up discussion (e.g. in a clinic waiting room, etc.).

The respondents also noted that they had used the series with groups of girls, boys, and with mixed groups (boys and girls). In addition, a few respondents had reportedly used the series with adults—parents, teachers and health workers.

Like *You, Your Life, Your Dreams*, the *Stepping Out* series was rated highly—4.2 out of 5. Respondents indicated that the issues covered in the series were highly relevant (4.6) and that the information was culturally appropriate (4.3). One respondent noted that "*Stepping Out* has covered almost all of adolescent issues, e.g. those in secondary schools, colleges, and school dropout" and another commented, "It is a very live example of what is happening in the community, so when shown to parents they will have a good way forward to advise their children."

The modules covering sexual health, unwanted sex and the changes that happen during puberty were cited as "most useful" by respondents, and most respondents reported that no modules were "least useful." Generally, respondents appeared to appreciate the overall format and style of the video, and especially the personal testimonies from young people and the interviews with adult experts and role models, which were rated 4.7. The music was the lowest rated aspect of the video (3.7).

The discussion guide was rated particularly highly in terms of its overall usefulness (5) and the clarity/easy-of-understanding of the instructions (4.5), however, one respondent wrote that "one needs to be serious and attentive to succeed. It become easier with several trainings. It gives a scare. It looks quite heavy on first impression—also is heavy."

The role plays outlined in the discussion guide were the most highly-rated activity (4.5), compared to the questions for discussion and other group exercises (e.g. values clarification exercises, quizzes, etc.), which were rated 4. However, one respondent noted that overall, the "questions, group exercises, and role-plays encourage adolescents to participate actively during the sessions." Other comments on the activities and learning approaches used in the series included: "teaching methodology is appropriate for adolescents and large groups" and that "group discussion is better because there is exchange of ideas, and learning from each other. Role plays helps someone not to forget."

Respondents offered a few suggestions for changing or modifying the *Stepping Out* series. For example, one individual suggested that additional female role models be presented in the second video module, which is focused on self-esteem, goal-setting and planning for the future. Another suggestion was that substance abuse be addressed more explicitly in the series. Finally, it was pointed out that the video series did not depict examples of good communication between young people and their parents, aunts or uncles, and it was noted that "It would be helpful for kids to see a positive response from adults because they clearly don't think that's what is to be expected."

In-depth Interviews

To support the written feedback gained through the evaluation questionnaires, the project partners conducted a series of in-depth interviews with users of the materials, and, as available, members of the target audiences with whom the materials have been used—namely adolescents and gatekeepers, such as parents, teachers, health workers and others who play an influential role in young people's access to reproductive health information and services.

Interviews and focus group discussions were conducted in Ghana, Kenya and Uganda. A series of open-ended questionnaires were developed to guide the interviews/focus group discussions conducted with each of the following audiences:

- **Facilitators—peer educators, youth workers, counselors, health workers and other program staff**: This questionnaire covered both materials—*Stepping Out* and *You, Your Life Your Dreams*—for those who are directly using the materials in their ongoing work with young people or others in the community.

- **Adolescents**: Two questionnaires were developed to solicit young people's feedback on the materials through interviews and/or focus group discussions. One interview guide was developed for use with young people who attended a session organized around *Stepping Out*, and another for interviewing adolescents who had read part or all of the information handbook, *You, Your Life, Your Dreams*.

- **Gatekeeper audiences, such as parents, teachers, health workers and other adults**: This questionnaire was designed to solicit feedback on the *Stepping Out* series from various gatekeepers who have attended a sensitization session using the materials.

Respondents included 20 facilitators (i.e. program staff and those who have led educational sessions or activities using *You, Your Life, Your Dreams* or *Stepping Out*). In addition, focus group discussions were held with adolescents (i.e. members of the target audience) and interviews and focus group discussions were conducted with representatives of secondary audiences (i.e. parents, teachers, health workers, etc.). Key findings related to each resource are presented below.

A. You, Your Life, Your Dreams

Interviews revealed that *You, Your Life, Your Dreams* is being used primarily as a reference material, though it is also used as a counseling tool; as a model for lesson plans and group discussions; and it is made available to young people at youth centers, clinics and schools. Several respondents reported using the book to train peer educators in reproductive health issues, and one said that it was used as the basis for dialogue in a radio show on reproductive health issues (see Annex II). Finally, several of those interviewed noted that they used the book as a personal reference ("I also use it in my own life as reference in making choices.").

Overall, program staff were extremely positive about the book's value as a reference or resource. Comments included

- "This book has made me more and more organized. It has improved my confidence during discussions because I have reference for anything I am not sure of.
- "This book has made me more systematic, especially in the discussions. It has enriched me with knowledge.
- "The book has actually improved my performance competencies. I am more organized in my discussions with young people. It enables me to prepare sessions.

- "The book is now our Bible for reference in counseling sessions for youth and in answering questions from youth."

Program staff were very positive about the book's impact and appeal for young people. One said that the book "helps youth clients who come to us to know that they are not alone in the situations depicted in the book. Usually they go away more confident about their sexuality or problems." Another noted that, "because it has details and is culture sensitive, the book has the capacity to promote positive sexual behavior. It can greatly impact [young people's] knowledge."

Respondents also appeared to value the various ways through which information, advice and facts are conveyed through the book—namely the book's cartoons/illustrations, "Did You Know" boxes chapter summaries, and quotes from young people about their own experiences and perspective on adolescence. The "Did You Know" boxes and the quotes from young people were most commonly cited as useful because they present the facts and offer peer perspectives on adolescence. One respondent noted that the "Did You Know" boxes "remove myth, enable one to explore and look for his/her concern areas and get questions answered." Another commented that these boxes provide useful answers to many adolescents' anxieties and unanswered questions."

A few respondents who were using the book solely as a reference material commented that the book's illustrations and cartoons were not useful. However, those who shared the book with young people reported that the artwork facilitated young people's understanding and contributed to their enjoyment of the book.

When asked which topic or chapter is most useful and important, facilitators' answers varied according to their areas of work and the needs of the youth with whom they work. One facilitator cited topics such as decision-making, relationships and "saying 'no'" as most important, whereas another reported that the chapter on emotional health and well-being ("Taking Care of Your Heart and Your Head") was one of the most important chapters: "Young people have never seen anything like this or been taught that things such as self-esteem exist."

The chapter on pregnancy and contraceptives was also cited as useful because it addresses many of the myths the youth hold. One respondent commented: "Many books deal with how you get pregnant, but most of them don't talk about the consequences of early pregnancy." He noted that *You, Your Life, Your Dreams* gets young people to "think about their lives and their futures."

Most program staff commented that no chapters were "least useful/ not important", however, a few acknowledged that they have had difficulty incorporating certain chapters into their programs. Chapter 13, focused on drugs and alcohol, was mentioned in this regard—e.g. "To me, all chapters are extremely useful except for 13, which we don't use quite often because that [issue] is not in our operation scope."

Most of those interviewed indicated that they would share the book with anyone, without hesitation, however, a few stated that the sections on condom use, contraceptives, safer sex and masturbation were controversial, with some saying that they always or frequently omitted these topics from discussion. One respondent explained that, "many [of those with whom he has shared the book] felt the tone of the book implies that it is all right to use condoms." He went on to explain that "sometimes you must go against what you feel and work with the people; otherwise you alienate yourself from the community and you get nowhere." Another commented that, "the chapters on condom use will upset many people but it is still important that this information is included."

Another facilitator commented that he would not use the book with religious leaders because "some will not agree with masturbation as a risk-free option for adolescents," and religious leaders "believe in abstinence and nothing else, and would therefore disagree also with any form of contraception for the unmarried." Another teacher/educator noted that he always skips the section on masturbation because it is "quite upsetting" and "just too controversial."

Despite the fact that the topic of masturbation is controversial, several facilitators voiced appreciation for its inclusion in the book. One noted that "Masturbation is not good but we need to have the information about it and [it is] not culturally inappropriate." Another respondent, who is a chaplain and school counselor in Nairobi, commented that the inclusion of masturbation in *You, Your Life, Your Dreams* gives it greater legitimacy as an alternative to sex. Observing that "most of the resistance to talking about sex and sexuality has been because there have been no alternatives," he recommended "If you broach the subject by talking about safe alternatives, you do not get resistance." Using *You, Your Life, Your Dreams* as a reference, this respondent said that he had held a conference with community parents and religious leaders to talk about homosexuality and masturbation, and he felt that since then, all the topics in the book have been accepted by the parents in his parish.

Like the adults interviewed, adolescents cited a wide variety of chapters as most interesting and useful. Recurring favorites with adolescents were the chapters focused on the changes adolescents go through during puberty, relationships, and emotional health and well-being. In a focus group discussion, one young person commented, "I learnt that all people my age are going through the same things I am going through. My situation is not peculiar and it is just a passing thing; I will grow out of it." Another said that she "learnt to be the driver of her own life and how to set goals and achieve them."

The adolescents interviewed were also enthusiastic about sharing the book with their parents—particularly the chapter, "Getting Along With Your Parents." One adolescent commented, "I would share this book with my parents because for years I have been trying to get them to understand me. So far I have not succeeded. When topics about relationships arise, it's war. I just feel this book will allow us to reach a compromise on certain issues." Another noted that parents "have something to learn from the book."

Adolescents also reported that the book was one that they would like to share with their friends. Several noted that they would share Chapter Nine ("Sex and Sexuality"). As one young person commented: "It seems that most of my friends and I have different ideas about pre-marital sex. All efforts to at least get to them to use condoms prove futile. I believe with the help of this book I will be able to get through to them because this book makes things clearer than I am able to make them. It's got more facts and examples, and moreover, it's not the mere words of an age-mate."

Adolescent respondents also appreciated the quotes from young people that are included throughout the book, saying that it is "important to reflect the thoughts of the young people." One respondent commented, "I like the quotes from other adolescents because I felt that this book was not only written by a couple of adults who wanted to impose their ideas on us again like always, but other adolescents were consulted for their views. I know we are on the same level and we understand each other better." Another reflected on the variety of perspectives reflected in the quotes: "It makes you gather views from people with different backgrounds and it helps."

Other features of the book, such as the illustrations/cartoons, glossary, and "Did You Know" boxes and chapter summaries, were also rated highly by adolescents. One focus group participant commented that "if an illiterate adolescent takes the book, though he cannot read, he can at least learn from the cartoons and illustrations." Adolescents agreed that the book was easy to understand and relevant to young people. One adolescent in the focus group discussion said, "[The book] is very educative and will help clear issues well. I believe it will prevent adolescents seeking advice which may be false from their friends."

Interviews with adults, such as parents, teachers, and health workers, indicated that the book also resonates with these "gatekeepers" and is a useful tool to sensitize these audiences about the issues facing adolescents. Several teachers commented that they learned a great deal from the book, and one noted that "The book created a lot of awareness in me. The main thing is how to help adolescents cope with some of the challenges that face or will face them." She reported that she had "learnt to be more appreciative of the needs of adolescents. [She] used to be more impatient with them before reading the book."

A school counselor interviewed during the evaluation reported that he had been providing training to the teachers in his school using both *Stepping Out* and *You, Your Life, Your Dreams*. The book is now being used as part of the school curricula and copies are kept in the library. This respondent reported that the book is very popular and that there has been " a big rush" to borrow the copies. Students have read the book "over and over" and the school librarian has to check each copy when it is returned in order to ensure that no pages are missing.

Almost none of those interviewed—program staff; adolescents or adults—offered any suggestions for strengthening or improving the book. A few program staff commented that sexual and reproductive rights should be explicitly addressed, and one commented that more detailed advice should be given to help young people seek help when problems arise (e.g. pregnancy, sexual assault, etc.). The most common suggestion was that the book have additional illustrations, and that the illustrations be enlarged and colored.

In conclusion, the interviews revealed that like *Stepping Out*, *You, Your Life, Your Dreams* is highly valued by youth and youth-serving staff alike for its comprehensive content and its culturally sensitive approach to adolescence and sexuality. Peer educators, teachers and others who work with adolescents, are using the book extensively but equally important, it also resonates with young people themselves. As one adolescent commented: "This book covers most if not all the topics that are of interest to people of my age. The truth is my secret question was answered by this book and I believe a lot of questions people of my age have, are well answered in this book as well."

B. Stepping Out

The *Stepping Out* series is being used in a variety of ways with many different target audiences; program staff reported that they use the set with in-school and out-of-school adolescents, urban and rural youth, peer educators, teachers, parents and health workers. Peer education programs, church groups, scout groups, youth centers and clinics are using the series. Generally, it appeared that the series is primarily used with adolescents, aged 14 to 24, however, some respondents working in urban areas reported using it with younger adolescents and children (aged 8 to 13), as well as with adults.

Feedback from program staff indicated that the series is a flexible health education tool that lends itself to many different uses. For example, some respondents reported that they use the series as it was originally designed—i.e. they show one video module to a small group of young people (ranging from 3 to 20 participants) and then conduct a follow-up discussion using the role plays, discussion questions, group exercises, etc. that are outlined in the *Stepping Out* discussion guide. Other respondents reported that they show modules to larger groups, primarily in schools (e.g. groups ranging from 50 to 300 young people), and lead their own discussion and "Question & Answer" session, without drawing on the activities and exercises outlined in the *Stepping Out* discussion guide. These respondents generally reported that they found it difficult to use the discussion guide with large groups—feedback that is not surprising, given that the set was specifically designed for use with small groups of no more than 20. As one respondent noted, "50 to 100 is a big group. Some do not see very well, and discussion becomes difficult to manage." Another commented: "Sometimes, during school visits, they are as many as 100 to 300. Usually there are too many discussions, and we cannot effectively control. Some questions end up being not answered and role plays become very difficult."

In contrast, program staff who are using the series with small groups reported that the video and discussion guide activities worked well together. The main feedback from these users was that they often lacked sufficient time to go through all the exercises and activities for each module. One respondent commented: "All the activities work well, except that we usually have limited time with young people to do all of them, as we want." Another noted: "You may have to choose more of other [exercises] and less of some due to time constraints.... We only used the role play and to me, it was working out perfectly well since it prompted the youth to open up and discuss issues. The discussions are also very useful."

Respondents also reported that they have adapted the series for different community needs. For example, one group of peer educators reported that they do puppet shows in schools and communities based on ideas, topics and the dialogue in the *Stepping Out* video. After using the puppet show to attract an audience, they screen the video and conduct a follow-up discussion. Because very large numbers of people of all ages tend to attend these community-level talks (e.g. 600 or more people), the peer education program reported that they divide participants by age and/or gender for the follow-up discussions.

Interestingly, while the video was primarily developed with an audience of urban and semi-urban youth as a target audience, some of those interviewed have been using the series with rural youth. These staff noted that rural adolescents have some difficulty understanding the accents of those who appear in the film and that rural youth are not well-represented in the film. These weaknesses notwithstanding, respondents stated that the issues covered in the video—relationships, HIV/AIDS, etc.—are extremely relevant for young people in rural areas. One user commented: "To a small extent, it does not depict the rural situation of young people, but even with this limitation it is quite useful." Respondents emphasized that the language of the film was very simple and clear, and that the way that the interviews, dramas and testimonies throughout the video are effective in that they appeal to people's emotions and serve as a catalyst for good discussions, despite socio-economic differences between rural youth and those featured in the film.

Overall, users' feedback was unanimously positive about the strengths of the series and its usefulness for structuring an educational session and stimulating discussion. Feedback included:

- "It helps me to direct the discussion to the specific topic because the students are focused on what they have seen."

- "The modules increase my confidence in discussing with the youth and even the parents."

- "The video has been very useful. Sometimes it says better what I would have wanted to bring out. In the same way, it provokes even quiet youth to talk."

- "It makes discussions with young people very active. It prompts them to ask questions. It makes it easy for the young people to interpret, understand and believe what we have been discussing all the years before. It provides confirmation and provides some answers beforehand."

- "The film is very stimulating, entertaining and educative. It promotes the youth to open up, forget their barriers and express themselves. They relate to the experiences of young people in the film."

- "It has been easy to use it because it has brief modules, [and the] use of testimonies from young people make the young people watching to believe the message. The language used is simple and words clear."

- "It is real. It makes young people believe the information therein. It motivates them to learn and stimulates questions."

There was little consensus among program staff regarding which of the video modules was most useful or relevant, and it appeared that most tailor their use of the series to the particular audience with whom they are working. For example, a facilitator working with teen mothers said that she found that Module Four (focused on unsafe abortion, sexually transmitted infections and HIV/AIDS) resonates among the girls she counsels, particularly the section on unsafe abortion. Representatives from another peer education program in Kenya noted that if all their youth workers were interviewed, every module of the video would be identified as "most critical" by at least one person.

Some of the peer education programs that are working with schools and conducting health talks and education sessions in schools noted that they find the second module ("What Do You Want To Be"), which focuses on goal-setting, self-confidence, self-esteem, etc., to be particularly useful and popular with school groups. As one program manager and counselor in Nairobi noted: "Hearing young people talk about their future and hearing others reach out and say you can succeed gives young people hope." Similarly, a youth worker involved with Maasai youth commented: "It really resonates with youth in high school—these youth are just starting to get jobs and think long-term."

The third module, "What Do You Mean By Love," was also cited as very popular among adolescents, because of its focus on peer relationships and relationships with parents. One user commented that some young people resist the notion that there is any kind of love other than sexual love, and that this module of the video is useful in stimulating discussion about this topic. Several facilitators noted that this module's focus on parent-child communication makes it particularly salient because this is a serious problem that many programs are trying to address through their work with both adolescents and their parents. One respondent reported that this module was used to help youth understand how to be both assertive and respectful—i.e. to communicate with their parents in a way that shows respect, but allows them to get their point across: "They learned what they can say to their parents and how to say it." Another facilitator reporting having shown this module several times to a group of peer educators in training: "The young people have even asked to borrow the video or stay late so they can watch the module again."

Respondents were also especially positive about the fifth module of the series, "Your Right To Say No", reporting that it always generates interesting and lively discussions. One user reported that this module "gave them good lessons" and helped clarify boys' misperceptions that when girls say "No" they actually mean "Yes." Another commented that "Youth, especially the girls, really respond to the sections on assertiveness and assertive behavior," and that "there is usually very good discussion about whether 'No' means 'No.' "

While the first five modules of the video were all cited by various respondents as most useful and well liked, it appeared that few of those interviewed found the last module ("Respect Yourself") to be particularly useful. As one youth worker noted, "We ask the youth to choose [which module they want to see], and they rarely select it." Another noted that they use this module least because they work primarily with younger adolescents who would not understand it. A third respondent reported that this module was not applicable to their work.

Feedback from adolescents and other secondary target audiences corroborated the feedback from program staff, rating the third and fourth modules ("What Do You Mean By Love?" and "Take Care and Be Safe") particularly highly. Several adolescents commented that they learned a lot about HIV/AIDS and STI prevention, noting that before seeing the video they had many misconceptions about STIs and HIV/AIDS: One commented: "At first I thought mosquitoes could spread AIDS but after watching the video, I know that mosquitoes cannot spread the disease." Other comments included: "On that day I learned that not all sexually transmitted diseases are transferred through sex. We can get it through sharing the same razor with an infected person" and "We were also taught to be good to our friends who have the AIDS virus. We should not neglect them. We should be good to them."

Adolescents were also positive about the fourth module, particularly the section of this module that deals with parent-child communication. Several adolescents said that this portion of their video was their favorite and that they would like their parents to see it. One adolescent explained: "The parents should call family meetings and talk. There is no

      Culture, Entertainment and Health Promotion

communication in the home. I think if parents watch, it will really help them." Another commented, "I think families should get the video so that they can sit to discuss the issues. They can also talk about HIV." All adolescents in the focus group say that they would recommend the video series to their friends, and one participant noted that if more young people could watch the video, "It would help them pass on the message on to other friends and the message will be spreading."

Interviews with parents and other secondary audiences, such as teachers, indicated that this module—and specifically the focus on parent-child communication problems—resonated with these groups as well. One parent commented that the module "really brought out the realities we face in our homes as far as communication with our children is concerned." Another said, "I learnt a lot. Most of the time, I don't listen to my children. I just want them to do what I like so I learnt something from the video." Some parents also noted that they planned to make changes in the ways they dealt with their children. For example, one person commented: "Number one, I am determined to go for walks with my children but it hasn't been possible. I want to make it possible and number two, I'm more sensitive to the things they tell me. I'm also determined to listen to my wife."

Parents who had watched the series were enthusiastic about having their children exposed to *Stepping Out*, and they agreed that it should be shown to fathers, mothers, teachers, and health workers—"everyone in contact with the youth."

Most of those interviewed—program staff and representatives of the target audiences—had relatively few suggestions for improving *Stepping Out*. One of the most common suggestions from facilitators, however, was that the modules be recorded on separate tapes because it is difficult to forward the video past modules that are not being shown As one respondent commented: "When one wants to show only one or a few of the modules, there is difficulty when the students are curious and insist on seeing other modules as well, which creates disappointment at times."

While one facilitator commented that the video is an "eye opener" for parents ("There is no better lesson for parents than this."), others suggested that the video would be better suited for adult audiences if it depicted "good parenting"—i.e. offered role models for parents. Some of the program staff interviewed had used the series with parents and other adult audiences, and reported that the video was useful in helping these audiences to overcome embarrassment and discomfort related to adolescent sexuality. Others suggested that a similar video series should be developed specifically for adults, such as parents, community leaders, church elders, etc. One respondent commented, "Visual aids will help them know that these problems of young people are real and that the way adults treat them dictates the choices they make in problems—e.g. abortion by young is a choice they make for fear of teachers and parents." Parents interviewed during the evaluation also suggested that featuring more adult scenes would help to emphasize to parents that "they have an important role to play in the life of their children during adolescence."

Other suggestions for improving the series focused primarily on depicting rural youth better and translating the dialogue into other local languages and dialects to improve understanding of the video content. One respondent noted that the series focuses more on girls than on boys, and that better role models should be presented for boys: "Boys should be depicted in a situation where they are educating others on the adolescent reproductive health needs of girls—e.g. there should be a boy emphasizing that girls' 'No' means 'No.' "

In sum, the interviews revealed that the *Stepping Out* series is being used extensively, with a variety of audiences in different contexts. Some of the staff interviewed commented that the series is the **only** tool they have to guide their health education, counseling and outreach efforts.

Clearly, programming work is being undertaken in order to deal with interpersonal and intergenerational dialogue.

Things to ponder about:

Africa has been misrepresented either consciously or unconsciously. The media has been accused of not being balanced. Clips screened also misrepresent Africa. Most of them have been shot in cities and can be seen to represent a whole spectrum of countries. But can the rural folk identify with the clips? This is a challenge to producers in urban environments.

- Great content is being produced. But is it reaching the unreached? This is a challenge. For example, are producers doing enough in terms of advocacy for public service? Television in Africa will continue to be a middle class item and therefore if one has a television programme, it means the target is the urban and peri - urban areas. Rural video may be an answer to the rural folk.

- There is need to consider a multi media approach in disseminating information since each medium has its own limitations. Let us consciously think about the alternatives and network amongst ourselves.

- Voicing of the voiceless is an important part of what everyone is trying to do particularly for young people who can have a forum. Sometimes we go to the youth with our own preconceived problems and impose them on the youth. We have to be careful so that the youth do not switch off. Let us think of how to empower these young people to script and produce their own programmes.

- With regard to the intergenerational communication, there is a split in communication between the young and the old. There is need to understand the competition say on FM Stations in East Africa and medium wave. The youth want information presented lightly and in this form. Let us seek an understanding of what the youth are listening to and what they are saying. We have to break cultural barriers between young and old. The only way to get to the youth is by acting and being like them. The good thing though is that younger producers are getting somewhere with the youth. Their capacity in dealing with the issues of the day needs to be enhanced

- It is difficult to describe how young people respond to all sorts of challenges. It is moving to submit to the hopelessness of Africa because a lot is happening on the ground. For example, Southern Africa has excelled in the arts and we should focus on some of the successes. We should learn from others.

- There is a lot of talent coming from Africa. We need to focus on what new history can be created by all this material coming from the youth.

- Let us distinguish between weeping and purposeful remembering in order to know where we are coming from and where we are going. If we do not understand our history and know what went wrong, then we cannot correct ourselves. There is no linking without yesterday. Unfortunately, many younger people think history is irrelevant.

- Most journalists swear in the name of freedom of press but most of them are questioning the content of our media. There is a magazine known as Red Paper that lobby groups have been advocating for its ban. As media practitioners do we not have a responsibility to lobby for censorship that is disseminated by media? Do we also lack creativity; for example is Channel O not a duplicate of MTV? How do we factor in ethics?

VIII

Art and History

Talking with young people nowadays, one gets the feeling that history is no longer important to them. Somehow, someone has convinced them that "history is dead." They are a generation that lives in the present; the past is unattractive, the present is sexy. But where does the inspiration for artistic creativity come from? How does one stand without a ground? The history of communities – their struggles with forces within and without; their hopes and aspirations; their disappointments – are all part of what informs their current state. Is it possible to ignore the narratives of communities in entertainment-education interventions? Can we erase the past and pretend it never existed? How do we ensure that re-membering of our dis-membered past is a reaffirmation of our humanity? How does one make artists remember not to forget where they came from? These questions are pertinent and we sought to think about them.

(The panelists included Gichora Mwangi of Karamu Trust, Kenya; Dr. Elizabeth Orchardson of Kenyatta University, Kenya and Michael Kawooya of Central Broadcasting Service (CBS FM Radio) Kampala, Uganda. John Molefe, of Soul City, chaired the session.)

Elizabeth Orchardson began by pointing out that her thoughts would focus more on questions rather than answers as a way of pinpointing the importance of art in the making of histories.

She said:

"The outcry over the looting of art museums in Iraq just a few months back is a timely reminder of the importance of art in world civilizations. The looting of Iraq art objects has destroyed the visual historical record of the Iraq people. It is the artifacts that over time have told the history of Iraq as the cradle of civilization; as the cradle of science, astronomy, and mathematics. Inscribed Iraq tablets, which were either looted or destroyed by American 'smart' bombs, were the historical records of the earliest form of writing in the world.

According to Jan Vansina "History without works of art remains bloodless, unreal…" (1984:196). Vansina further says, "we cannot assume that art is unimportant in general historical reconstructions, whether in Africa or elsewhere." (1984:196)

A Japanese scholar, Umasao Tadao, notes that in Japan "… people have noticed the value of everyday objects. They have come to see the importance of preserving such objects. And they have begun to think of history itself as the accumulation of everyday objects" and that "Museums are a civilization's institutions or record (2001:10-11)."

The historical development of art is often inevitably linked to the socio- economic development of human society. For example, with the development of the feudal system in Europe with its definite class divisions, art was increasingly seen as a capable of visually symbolizing the aspirations of the ruling class. Art subjects such as painting, sculpture and architecture were used as powerful tools to propagate the supremacy of the feudal class ideology."

Elizabeth Orchardson went on to argue for people to seek knowledge:

"We in Africa have often been very dismissive of art and its importance. This is partly due to ignorance and under-exposure to art. As a result, we have failed to see the importance of art in the construction of African history. How many of us are aware of the rock art of Sub-Saharan and Saharan Africa? The rock paintings can be deconstructed to give us an understanding of human and animal presence and activities, technologies, and materials. For instance, the materials used testify to the African technology of pigment and binder preparation and use. These ancient pigments have survived for thousands of years. Rock art is thus a valuable contribution in the history of technology or the science of pigments and binding agents.

The 'Nok Culture' of West Africa is an example of an iron technology center which flourished in about 500 B.C to 200 A.D (Vansina, 1984). Nok is believed to have produced iron in smelting furnaces (Gillon, 1984:86). In addition, the Nok people produced life-sized clay sculptures which were fired and which have survived.

In Ethiopia, we have the rock-hewn churches of Lalibela and Gondar. An example is the Abba Lebanos in Lalibela, which was carved out of live rock. It is dated to A.D. 119 - 1225 (Gillon). The church is 9 meters high x 7 meters x 7 meters. The most incredible aspect of these rock-hewn churches is the technology used. The live rock was carved away in the same way that a subtractive sculpture is created. These churches reproduced all the elements of European basilicas such as beams, lintels, arches, and so forth. It is mind-boggling to imagine that architects and carvers could visualize a building and genius and dedication behind these monumental works of art. I would like to suggest that we need to view these Ethiopian churches as the repositories of African intellectual genius and history. Fortunately, these churches were not able to be excavated and carried away to Western museums!

Elsewhere in Africa, we have other civilizations whose art of objects have contributed to the making of African history. The art of West Africa is well-documented and its place in history is generally well-acknowledged. In Eastern Africa, we have the architecture of the Swahili and the ruins of the Great Zimbabwe. The people of Great Zimbabwe were experts in mining and building. In the 13th century A.D., building in stone began. Structures such as the Colonial Tower and the Elliptical Building were constructed out of granite block without the use of mortar. The buildings were extensive in diameter and height.

Nubia has long been described as the cradle of Sub-Saharan art (Gillon 1984:55). By the time of the Early Dynastic Period in Egypt, starting about 2955 BC, the indigenous at of Nubia was already well developed. The city of Meroë of ancient Nubia is an outstanding example of African historical fact. Meroë is often described by historians as "the Birmingham of ancient Africa" because of its iron technology (Sayce, 1911:55) In addition, Meroitic architects designed and produced impressive buildings, some of which have survived as ruins.

There are many other examples of the importance and influence of art throughout Africa. My concern is that we have not appreciated this vital contribution. Unfortunately, because of our Euro-centri and Ameri-centri education, attitudes and influence, many of us seem unable to appreciate the richness and diversity of our African heritage and legacy. Our schools do not teach our children the greatness of places such as

Nok, Meroë, Great Zimbabwe, Benin, etc. (when I was in primary school I could name all the great rivers, mountains, our countries of Europe and America and knew very little about Africa). In the contemporary times we seem caught up with trying to be more British than the British and more American than the Americans. We overlook our own greatness, our own potential. And in the process we distort history and historical fact. Art is seen as unimportant. Yet, in the Western World Act is viewed as the very foundation of their civilization. We have buried our own history under the debris of western history and cultures. Colonialism largely denied the existence of African art and we have continued the tradition of denial. Art objects, as demonstrated by our so-called traditional art object, represent the creativity and genius of Africa and help to establish a historical record of our achievement, yet we don't seen to appreciate these facts.

How many of our soap operas make use of African visual art - both ancient and modern background, costumes, etc?

We in Kenya, need to appreciate the recent decision by the Kenyan Government to stop the exportation of the Murumbi Collection to Britain. This said, how many of us knew or know about this valuable collection? How many of us know that the other Murumbi Collection housed at the National Archives was bought by the Kenyan Government, in 1977, together with the former Murumbi House in Muthaiga for Kshs. 6.3 million? How many of us know that the house was later grabbed by a well-connected personality, pulled down and another mansion constructed in its place? If we do not know those facts, how can we recognize the importance of art in the making of history?" she concluded.

Elizabeth Mazrui, by urging us to seek art and to be more appreciative of it is reaffirming the relationship between human beings and creativity. Through art we are able to rediscover ourselves and our environment. Art fulfils two functions: the *dulce* (aesthetics) and *utile* (utility). By oscillating within those domains, art can make us better human beings.

In order to get a practitioner's view, we sought the CBS, Uganda. Its manager,

Michael Kawooya Mwebe, began by defining entertainment as a piece of performance involving music, dance, drama, and literature that is meant to amuse people. Art is a form of entertainment, which incorporates music, dance, drama, and history as an account of events as they happened in the past.

He then raised the question of what constitutes African histories and went on to say that in the book *Come Back*, Leroy E. Mitchelle JR. (1988) made extensive research about he African visual histories: He wrote:

> "The Sahara can be called the largest museum in the world. From Egypt across the continent to the Atlantic are frescoes on rocks and caverns done as early as 10,000 B.C picturing African people dancing, farming, hunting and performing everyday tasks. Elegant costumes and masks are also portrayed, and most of these relics are still worn by tribes throughout tropical Africa. Because the budding cities of tropical Africa are slowly destroying and modifying the ancient relics, the correlation between the ancient and the recent must be made, and made soon."

According to Kawooya:

"Mitchell goes ahead to highlight other aspects of African visual history which include dress, habits, styles, masks, painting and culture.

However, in his work, Mitchelle makes an oversight of the oral aspects of African histories which include story telling, traditional and folk songs (music), proverbs and parables most of which made a reflection of the socio-economic, culture and political ways of life of the African people. The few aspects of African history reflected clearly demonstrate that it was dominated by art which reflected a whole complete society.

Why did art play a dominant role in the shaping of African History? It is because it was the most effective means of communication and mobilization, its level of development/technology, its literacy levels, and its source of motivation and inspiration.

Amilcar Cabral in a paper presented at the Ugandan British High Commission during a workshop on culture in 1987 said "culture is simultaneously the fruit of a peoples history by the positive of negative influence it exerts on the evolution of relations between man and his environment and among men or human groups with society as well as between different societies".

Looking at drama as a form of art and as a culture, it evolves ideas, issues and themes from one individual to another, one society to another and from generation to generation. Drama as an art is one decent form of entertainment which talks so much about our past and present.

It is through this form of art that individuals can ably communicate to the masses, which yields a positive response and concise understanding issues regardless of whether the audience understands the language or not.

Art is an archive of great historical interest giving an essential first hand account on the developments of pre-and post independence Africa.For all this period art has recorded society's criticisms, comments, compliments, features and successes in different forms poetry, drama, music or novelty.

It is no longer fashionable to attend theatre only for purposes of fun or passing time. Nowadays people want quality entertainment that stimulates, excites and above all educates society. This implies that people prefer those pieces of art which appeal to the audience from all aspects of life and most importantly that adds value to their lives. In contemporary life, several institutions including NGOs and several sections of civil society have resorted to art to communicate important messages aimed at influencing and hence causing social change. In many African countries, this is done through drama, music and poetry.

In Uganda, following outbreak of the AIDS pandemic, the government in collaboration with local drama groups staged a play titled *NDIWULIRA* which made considerable impact in the sensitization of Ugandans on the dangers of HIV/AIDS. This partly accounts for Uganda's success story, by international standards, in controlling this pandemic.

Alex Mukulu, in his play *30 years of Bananas*, takes us through a satirical view of what Uganda benefited, suffered and lost over the three decades since independence. All this is done in 3 hours as told by one experienced refugee from Rwanda. This is not a story that can be told in just 3 hours, but because of drama, the artist entertains us as we learn what happened during and after the 30 years of independence.

Does art still have a significant role to play in Africa's present and future socioeconomic development programmes? The traditional ways of life are changing rapidly. Two hundred years of European interference, new socio-economic development ideologies and programmes and settlement have profoundly influenced the thinking, behaviour and perceptions of many Africans. The introduction of industries and spread of education have opened up new ways of thinking and earning a living. Each passing year, more and more people move from the countryside to the cities and towns in search of education and better jobs in factories and offices. However, many Africans are still reluctant to abandon the traditional rural way of life because of the security it offers. Those who do venture into the cities usually find great difficulties in getting employment and accommodation. Many African governments are not always able to meet the ever increasing demands of their people. The changes are not rapid and or smooth enough to satisfy people's demands. Economic and social dislocation, as well as political strife are often the result.

Africans now live in times of conflict where global trends are alienating them from their rich/valuable culture and heritage and hence forcing them to embrace mass culture. This has left Africans alienated, insulted, confused, bored and patronized. The recipients needs, interests feelings and concerns are usually not taken care of. The effectiveness of the communication processes has always been seriously reduced hence making little positive impacts.

The challenge before us today is to find out whether a mass culture is sustainable. Can we manipulate it to bring social change? This trend of events calls for a unique approach if governments, NGOs and civil society are to cause meaningful, positive and sustainable change in African societies. We ought to advocate for influencing population trends, and encouraging sustainable development by enhancing communication that is sensitive to national and local cultures of the target groups. This approach is not only unique but it also blends well the past with the present paving way for a smooth social-cultural and attitude change. In addition, the approach is appropriated as it respects human values and dignity thus conforming to the broadly accepted United Nations covenants and resolutions.

The CBS experience is a case for social programming/social marketing. CBS FM is the pioneer FM radio station in Uganda to make a deliberate effort to depart from copycat radio broadcasting which was simply lifting from the western radio forms. Nine years ago, tuning into any of the radio stations in Kampala, one would not tell whether the station was based in New York, London, or Amsterdam. It was evident that we had blindly and wholesomely succumbed to the mighty globalisation and mass culture. CBS set out on the un-beaten path and set the trend to the new African broadcasting philosophy. The station's guiding philosophy was and still is to use Buganda Kingdom's rich culture and heritage by blending it with the modern social ideological and technological advancements to mobilize and sensitize the people so as to influence their attitude and social welfare improvements. CBS programming is deliberately designed to reflect this philosophy. Dr. Hans Martin and his co-writer Bindanda M'pia in their book *"Natural Medicine in the Tropics"* emphasize the need for Africa to look within itself to heal itself from diseases.

CBS uses the arts as instruments of delivering messages based on scientific research. These messages are delivered using the language, formats and styles that are sensitive to our cultural values which are not only familiar with the listeners but are also appealing to the target audience.

The messages on the radio are intended to entertain, stimulate positive change, and most importantly, empower the individual. The recipients get inspired and motivated by these messages as they identify with their ways of life and are in a Luganda language - a local dialect which they fully understand and identify with.

The government of Uganda and other development agencies have recognized the significant role of CBS in economic and social change and it is on the basis of this recognition that CBS is a key partner in broadcasting for several development programmes.

CBS has been successful in developing a unique multimedia package which is used in Functional Adult Literacy Programmes in rural areas of Uganda. The package is a combination of drama, comic books, charts and a radio programme. This programme is done in conjunction with the government of Iceland.

CBS has been very instrumental in designing and disseminating educational messages in the fight against HIV/AIDS, rural sanitation, hygiene, protection of the environment, adopting profitable agricultural practices and civic education.

The role of CBS has gone far beyond broadcasting. They are partners and players at various levels of social development (nsidika njake). This explains the background to their business slogan "CBS your partner in development".

They started this idea by designing and broadcasting a programme called *NEKOLERA GYANGE* (literally translated as "I do my own business") which focuses on the small business sector and individual business practitioners. Now CBS is a key player in the organization of a more developed version of this concept *Business-to-Business exhibition"* which they have planned to be an annual event.

CBS is growing and attracting more and more partners in our deliberate efforts to use African culture and heritage as a vehicle for effective and positive socio-economic change in the present days of the Internet and Globalisation. They are not looking at these forces as a threat. On the contrary, their approach is aimed at the safe and smooth anchoring for the new ideological and technological advancements, mainly from the West, to the African setting without necessarily shocking and/or dislocating them. Earlier methods have been counter productive and can be proclaimed to be out of tune.

IX

Meeting Donor Expectations

A major challenge for entertainment education programs is funding. Although certain partners in the donor community now recognize the importance of entertainment-education interventions a lot of work remains to be done. It is, therefore, fitting to hear the voices of two people who have been supporting entertainment-education work in East Africa. The continued dialogue between 'those who give the money' and those who implement programs is vital if we are to make progress in using entertainment-education for social change. The dialogue allows for a negotiated position before, during, and after project implementation. We sought to hear from people who have been involved in grant making.

(The panelists were Mary Anne Burris, the then Program Officer-Reproductive Health, Ford Foundation and Rob Burnet the Program Officer- Media, Arts and Culture at Ford Foundation, Nairobi. The session was chaired by Kakai Karani of Jomo Kenyatta Foundation, Nairobi)

Maryann Burris said: "In my brief minutes on this panel about donor expectations I will simply raise three questions regarding the issue before us:

What story? (Which is about truth)? Who be Story? (Which is about agency) and what is a donor? (Which is about strategy and power).

In the tradition we have had thus far set out at the Summit, allow me to begin with a story.

I love school and I have a thirsty mind. Whenever I was not sure about the next step in my life, I would go back to school. My earlier degrees are all the humanities: literature, philosophy, folklore, languages were the stuff on my passion and pursuit. I spent one whole semester in graduate school studying the many birds mentioned in the Chinese poetic classic, the Shih Ching and matching their occurrences and stories, I buried my head in any depiction of the oracles and rituals of the Cheyenne and Comanche tribes, both running in my bloodstream. Anyway, these were the things I adored. But when I decided as an already over-thirty single mother to study towards a doctorate, my politics and activism compelled me. In fact, I hardly ever cared how they ended, so I had to force myself to read them through.

I had noticed that my anthropology of development professor often carried a book of poetry along with his texts and I decided to approach him to ask him if, indeed, I was in the wrong place. So I went to his office and spilled out my heartfelt fears that I had landed in the wrong place-the wrong field of study for me. Thinking that he would reassure me and tell me all the reasons why I was in the RIGHT place, I was surprised to hear him first say, " well, maybe you are in the wrong place. You see, you have a humanities heart and mind. This means that you find truth in the single instance- in the single breathtaking sunrise, in the single metaphor, in one woman's story, in a painting or dance. And your classmates and professors and the field you have entered can only see truth in the aggregate. They want proof in the collective, generalized hypothesis. This is where they find truth. And unless you can at least come to understand this truth as well, and become competent in assessing it, questioning it, accepting it, you will not succeed in this field of study."

I cannot tell you how this helped me. Because it meant that I did not have to reject my own way of seeing and feeling the truth, but I could learn another way; become bifocaled, as it were.

I tell this story to highlight the link that the activist artist makes between the individual truth, what Micere Mugo calls "our authentic word" in her poem, and what Kimani Njogu called "our collective efficacy" the aggregate truth- our aim to change society for the better. I also tell this story to underscore the notion what is most true to the donor in structural terms and what is true to the creative artist, the story itself, can find common land and language. And it must be only in those places where these two truths intersect, when telling the authentic story and hoping to use our power as storytellers, as activist, artists, overlap where we can meet one another's expectations. So, we look for those times when our two truths find consonance instead of shaping ourselves by the often-arrogant aim to change other people's minds and behaviors. And, as much as of the wonderful performance, video and radio stories we have shared attest, these places of honest consonance to exist and enliven our work at both ends.

How do we, when, do we meet donor expectation? When our truths can speak to each other. I can tell you that in my 13 years on the signing sides of the check- first in China and now in East Africa, my job as a donor has been to contribute to work that ensures women's rights, that promotes youth, that assures sexual health, that cares for the sick and encourages the young, that promotes solvent families- in short, that contributes to social change. And in resourcing media and artistic expression the basic rule of how to do that well is the same – it is all about agency. Whose story is it anyway? Does it express a truth that we should hear and acknowledge? Is it real? AGENCY.

The first question to ask is not how to meet donor expectations, but what are your own. Your own truth, your own story, and is there a common ground between that and the instrumental goal of a funder. Only when there is an authentic voice does the piper's tune meet the call of the payer, the musician and his audience. I wonder about the difference between having to meet the call of the message (donor) and the advertiser (the commercial). As Marvin Hanke said yesterday, first we must do good work.

The last question was about donors themselves, donors, ourselves I suppose I should say. For it is not until I moved to Kenya that I began to hear the dreaded word "donor" as if we constituted a species all our own. As if we all went to donor school to become something beside ourselves. While I am familiar with the position, nothing thus far said at this Soap Summit as in "Donors think culture is an obstacle to change... Donors don't recognize the difficulties of the artist...." Rings true to me, Mary Ann, one of the so-called "donors". My point is this; it is wise to have a nuanced understanding of the donor. I mean this in terms of both of the balance between the program person you partner with her foundation or agency, and in terms of differences between donors themselves- their definitions of success, their need for visibility, and their funding dynamics.

Rob and I work for a relatively progressive Foundation which has always recognized agency, which cannot raise money and therefore has little real need for its logo everywhere, and which funds in the arts directly- as expression as well as a player in social change. So, we are a bit typical. And, still, we have our mandate – among them to announce your "benchmarks of success" if you are to receive grant monies. These must match the programmatic areas of interest and strategies developed within the foundation itself to be funded.

This does not mean that Ford does not recognize that there is plenty of good and worthy effort which falls outside of these parameters. It simply means these are the rules. The more you can learn about this and share information with one another about these differences within the donor world, the better for your strategy. In some ways, all donor-supported efforts are part of globalization, which we have touched on from many angels. In some ways, who is a donor? We are all donors. We need certainly to broaden our vision about who is a potential backer of supporter of our work- from the audience to the community to the company. What local money, effort, enthusiasm can be brought on the donor role?

I can also say that after all these years as a donor, one of my most basic tenet for judging potential partners is whether or not they can say NO to money. Sometimes it is best just to say no. Stay true to the true story."

Rob Burnet gave brief comments. He said that he had hoped all those who had made presentations would have started theirs by examining the Summit's theme *Making Entertainment Useful* but none had. For him, the theme would have been better if it had recognized that entertainment is already useful and examine creativity as a way of exercising social change, giving a voice to the voiceless.

He pointed out that having value for creativity is different for donors. Creativity for society's sake is vital. Imagination is fed by having people tell their stories and is more important than knowledge. In producing Africa soaps, whose story is the producer telling (agency and ownership)? The only critical shape of the story comes down to who owns it. It is about quality of the story, ownership and the people telling it.

In terms of expectations, the greatest one we should have is that donors disappear. This has to do with sustainability and we need to discuss for example if it is possible for local television to be financed locally. We also need to discuss how to make donors meet our own creativity.

Things to ponder about:

- When working with donors, one has to produce drafts of effects and results, yet as producers we have done stories that have touched people's hearts. However, donors are not interested in this aspect of our work. How can we negotiate with them in order to emerge with a win – win situation?

- There are organizational structures that must demonstrate benchmarks of success. This is the language that needs to show certain power of change. Can this be done all the time?

- How does one measure effects and impact in the arts? Is it possible for partners to have faith that artists are actually doing the work they sought to do without necessarily giving quantifiable results?

- Most artists spend a lot of time writing proposals that will meet donor expectations at the expense of creativity. There is need to define the common objective between an artist and a donor. Capacity building among entertainment-education practitioners is equally vital and urgent.

- Art is dynamic and keeps changing. Usually a majority of artists write a proposal that has an exaggerated budget and therefore make it difficult for the donor to meet their expectations. Donors need to hold meetings with artists and explain what their expectations are. If this does not happen, funding will continue going to the wrong people who have perfected their lobbying skills. Artists are not good proposal writers. How can their skills be improved?

- There is simply not enough funding to go to everyone. For example, the Ford Foundation receives over 100,000 proposals yet only 2000 are funded every year. This makes it difficult to select and, therefore, the quality of the proposal matters. Most artists are left out because they cannot write creatively in their letter of intent. The truth is that those who know how to lobby end up getting the funding. There is a constant balance between risk, lack of words and creative writing. Minimum standards and language should go into the proposals as funding cannot be granted just for the sake of giving or because certain people are friends. However there are donors who are now accepting proposals written in any Kenyan language and handwritten for small grants. There is more dialogue taking place between those implementing projects and those funding.

- Trying to please the donor is a wrong approach. It should be about the 'agency' that is, whose idea is it? Is it what the proposal writer wants to achieve? This is a difficult and complex business. Donors try to read between the lines.

- Donors have guidelines and people have to answer certain questions. Foundations also have criteria and a strategy for grant making that will contribute significantly to changes on the ground. But great work will always be funded.

- Also as a way of building donor confidence in order to attract funding, there is, wealth in creative arts in this region and that it takes certain donors time to understand context.

X

Research, Monitoring and Evaluation

The evolution of entertainment-education is posing new challenges and providing some answers to earlier problems. In many cases, it is not quite evident in certain entertainment-education programs the theoretical underpinnings of the intervention. This absence of clarity right from the onset makes it difficult to determine the success or failures of the interventions. In any case, when there is no deliberate link between research and the program, the results of the evaluation may not be very useful and may not contribute in improving the program.

Similarly, results may impressive but would need to be pegged on specific interventions; a situation that may be cumber-some if it was not imagined.

A significant number of entertainment-education interventions are relying on Bandura's social cognitive theory. Briefly, the theory states that people lean behaviour, attitudes, and beliefs by observing models. In order to enhance the learning process, the attractive models are rewarded and the non attractive ones punished.

Thus a research agenda would need to look at how models influence behaviour among the target audience. One challenge with research is funding. Due to financial constraints, EE interventions in Africa are not well researched before, during and after the program. Because of the absence of monitoring and evaluation results in many Africa based entertainment-education programs, it becomes difficult to continue funding such initiatives because sponsors want to see the effects of the intervention. There is also the tension between continuing to produce non-monitored programs which intuitively are effective and spending most of the money on research. Apparently, the key is to create a balance between the two important activities. In order to reflect more systematically on research and programming we listened to the voices of reknown researchers.

(The panelists were Peter Vaughan of Minnesota and Arvind Singhal of Ohio University. The session was chaired by Marvin Hanke of Malawi).

Arvind Singhal made a presentation on *Integrating Entertainment-Education Broadcasts with Community Listening and Service Delivery in India: Lessons for Programming and Research*

"We listen to each episode of *Taru*. We then discuss the episode's content in our listeners' club. Through the medium of *Taru*, we are learning lots of new things, and I am trying to incorporate many of them in my life to make it better. After listening to this radio serial, we have taken decisions to wipe out the caste discrimination in our village, teach *dalit* (lower caste) children, and to pursue higher education." — Vandana Kumari, a 17 year-old member of Village Kamtaul's *Taru* listeners club, Bihar State, India, in a personal interview, September 2, 2002.

The young woman quoted above listens regularly to the radio serial, *Taru*, broadcast by All India Radio (AIR), the Indian national radio network. Her father, Shailendra Singh, is a rural health practitioner (RHP) in Kamtaul Village in Bihar State, and a respected public figure (in summer, 2002, he was elected a Ward Commissioner). Singh's health clinic is called a *Titly* (Butterfly) Center, and is part of a network of 20,000 rural health practitioners, organized by Janani, a non-governmental organization that promotes reproductive health care services in the poor Indian States of Bihar, Jharkhand, Madhya Pradesh, and Chattisgarh. These four States have a population of 190 million people; the highest fertility, infant mortality, and maternal death rates in India; and the lowest literacy and contraceptive prevalence rates.

In 1999, Shailendra Singh and his wife, Sunita, underwent a three-day course in reproductive health care, first-aid, maternal and child health, and diagnosis and treatment of STIs/RTIs (sexually-transmitted infections and reproductive tract infections) at a Janani training facility in Patna. Janani purposely invited both Singh and his wife for training as most rural Indian woman are embarrassed to seek reproductive health services from a male RHP. Now, with a trained woman health practitioner Sunita (referred by village women as *Didi* or "sister"), female villagers could discuss sex, seek prenatal and antenatal care, and access contraceptives. After registering in Janani's rural health network, Singh's clinic in Kamtaul Village began to stock Janani's branded *Mithun* ("Bull") condoms, *Apsara* ("Angel") oral contraceptive pills, and pregnancy dipsticks.

In February, 2002, Singh and Sunita's health practice in Kamtaul Village became the center of a novel experiment in entertainment-education radio broadcasting, when All India Radio, in cooperation with Population Communications International (PCI), New York, broadcast an entertainment-education radio soap opera *Taru* (the name of the program's female protagonist) in four Hindi-speaking states, Bihar, Jharkand, Madhya Pradesh, and Chhatisgarh. All India Radio and PCI's ground-based partner in these four Indian states was Janani. Pre-program publicity for *Taru* was conducted on-the-air by All India Radio and, on-the-ground, *Taru* was publicized by Janani's 20,000 strong network of RHPs (like Singh and Sunita), *Taru* posters, and over 700 strategically-placed wall paintings at major highway intersections (Singhal & Rogers, 2003).

In four villages in Bihar State, selected carefully to fulfill certain criteria (detailed later), folk performances dramatizing the Taru storyline were carried out (led by one of the present authors, Sharma) a week prior to the radio serial's broadcasts to prime the message reception environment. Shailendra Singh's Kamtaul Village was one such site for the folk performances. Singh and his wife Sunita spread word-of-mouth messages about the folk performance, encouraging hundreds of people to attend, and awarded transistors (with a sticker of Taru's logo) to groups who correctly answered questions based on the folk performance. These groups were then formalized as Taru radio listening clubs. Each group received an attractive notebook (with a Taru logo), and were encouraged urged to discus the social themes addressed in Taru, relate them to their personal circumstances, and record any decisions, or actions, they took as a result of being exposed to Taru.

RHP Shailendra Singh's daughter, Vandana, her younger sister, a cousin, and two friends formed the young women's listening club in Kamtaul Village. A *Taru* fever has since raged in the Singh household. Discussions of *Taru* inspired the Singh family to undertake several new initiatives: They stopped a child marriage in Kamtaul Village, launched an adult literacy program for *dalit* (low-caste) village women, and have facilitated the participation of *dalits* in community events. Further, since *Taru* began broadcasting, Singh's monthly sales of *Mithun* condoms and *Apsara* pills have jumped 400 percent.

What explains such ground-breaking social changes as are occurring in Kamtaul Village? The present paper argues that synergistic possibilities for social action can emerge when entertainment-education radio broadcasts are strategically integrated with community-based group listening and locally-available health care services. Social transformation was catalyzed when (1) All India Radio provided the entertainment-education "air cover" in the form of *Taru*, (2) *Taru* listening groups acted as informal organizing units for social deliberation and local action, and (3) Janani's rural health network provided the ground-based service delivery. Each component complemented the contribution of the other.

In the present paper, we provide a historical background on the *Taru* Project, a description of its on the air and on-the-ground components, and the radio serial's storyline. Our methodology for assessing the impacts of *Taru* is described, including the use of video testimony and participatory photography. We then present the results from our community-based study in certain select villages of Bihar State, explaining the process through which community members enact system-level changes as a result of exposure to *Taru*. We investigate the power dynamics, the resistances, and the audience members' struggles in the process of media-stimulated change, a process involving parasocial interaction, peer communication, and collective efficacy.

Historical Background: From *Tinka* to *Taru*

The inspiration for the *Taru* Project came from a previous community-based investigation of the impacts of *Tinka Tinka Sukh* (Happiness Lies in Small Pleasures), a radio soap opera, in Lutsaan Village of North India. In January, 1997, 184 villagers in Lutsaan signed a pledge not to give, or accept, dowry (an illegal but widespread social practice in India). These villagers also pledged to not allow child marriages (also an illegal but common practice), and pledged to educate daughters equally with their sons (Papa, Singhal, Law, Pant, Sood, Rogers, and Shefner-Rogers, 2000). Lutsaan villagers mailed the petition, in the form of a colorful 20 by 24 inch poster-letter, to All India Radio, which was broadcasting *Tinka Tinka Sukh*. In the radio program, a young woman, Poonam, is abused by her husband and his parents for bringing an inadequate dowry, until she commits suicide.

The poster-letter stated: "Listeners of our village [to "*Tinka Tinka Sukh*"] now actively oppose the practice of dowry – they neither give nor receive dowry." A young tailor in the village was especially influenced by the radio program episodes about dowry, and initiated the process of writing the poster-letter among the people in his tailor shop. As a result of the forces set in motion by the tailor, the villagers formed radio listening clubs, planted trees for reforestation, and built pit latrines for improving village sanitation. Girls' enrollment in the village's schools increased from 10 percent at the time of the radio broadcasts, to 38 percent two years later. Fewer dowry marriages and child marriages occurred in Lutsaan, although these practices did not disappear completely in the village (Papa et al., 2000).

Authors Singhal and Papa conducted an in depth case study of the empowerment process in Lutsaan over several years (Singhal & Rogers, 1999; Papa et al., 2000). The Lutsaan case study suggested entertainment-education interventions have their strongest effects on audience behavior change when messages stimulate reflection, debate, and interpersonal communication about the educational topic among audience members (Papa et al., 2000), and when services can be delivered locally. These insights from Lutsaan were applied in formulating the *Taru* Project, which included a partnership with a ground-based service delivery organization, Janani; pre-program publicity of *Taru* through Janani's extensive RHP network; and the establishment of listeners' groups to encourage peer-based conversations.

The *Taru* Project

Taru was a 52-episode entertainment-education radio soap opera, broadcast in India from February 2002 to February 2003 after a creative design workshop facilitated by Kimani Njogu, Susan Rhodes and Kate

Randolph. Its purpose was to promote gender equality, small family size, reproductive health, caste and communal harmony, and community development. *Taru* began broadcasting in Bihar, Jharkhand, Madhya Pradesh, and Chattisgarh States in India on February 22, 2002 (and later in the entire Hindi-speaking belt of North India from May, 2002). One episode was broadcast each week on Friday at 8:00 p.m., with a repeat broadcast each Sunday at 3:40 p.m. Each episode of *Taru* began with a theme song, and a brief summary of the previous episode. Each episode ended with an epilogue that posed a question to the listeners, inviting them to write-in their responses to AIR. Half-way through the *Taru* broadcasts (in October, 2002), Kiran Bedi, a well-known woman police officer in India and a social activist, hosted two interaction programs with *Taru's* listeners, answering questions on-the-air.

The idea of integrating on-air entertainment-education broadcasts with ground-based listening and service delivery, was floated in September, 2000, in a New York-based meeting between David Andrews and Kate Randolph of Population Communications International; Gopi Gopalakrishnan, Arisingh Dutt, and Shejo Bose of Janani; and author Singhal of Ohio University. As a first step, PCI hired MODE, an India-based research organization, to conduct a literature review and site-based formative research (in Bihar and Madhya Pradesh States) to distill the educational issues to be addressed in *Taru*. In the next 17 months, the *Taru* Project progressed rapidly, as roles and responsibilities of the partners were defined.

PCI looked after the overall management of the *Taru* Project: It provided the technical assistance for creating the radio serial, sponsored a visit for half-a-dozen members of All India Radio's creative team to Bihar State to gain familiarity with Janani's program, and hosted a workshop with the AIR creative team to design a blueprint for the radio serial. Ohio University (1) designed the Project's theoretical framework for integrating *Taru's* on-the-air and on-the-ground activities, (2) carried out a pre-test of *Taru's* pilot episodes in collaboration with the Center for Media Studies (CMS), New Delhi, and (3) implemented the summative research evaluation plan (detailed later) for the present project in collaboration with CMS. Janani sponsored the broadcasts of *Taru* in the four states, worked with Ogilvy Outreach, a Bombay-based advertising and PR agency, to develop a logo for *Taru* as well as the pre-program publicity materials (posters, stickers, flyers, and wall paintings), distributed these materials to RHPs, and provided logistical support to (a) Brij Lok Madhuri to conduct the *Taru* folk performances, and (b) to Ohio University and the Center for Media Studies to conduct the field-based research in Bihar State. All India Radio was responsible for producing the radio serial, broadcasting it, and for inviting and collecting listeners' feedback.

Researching *Taru*

Our research on *Taru* is guided by methodological triangulation, the use of multiple research methods (both quantitative and qualitative) to measure the same phenomenon. While the present paper relies primarily on data collected from a community case study of Village Abirpur in Vaishali District of Bihar State, and from our observations of Village Kamtaul, Madhopur, and Chandrahatti (where a high degree of field orchestration, including folk performances were conducted) in Bihar's Muzaffarpur District, other forms of data were collected to deepen our understanding of how *Taru* influenced its audience: (1) Personal interviews with key officials involved in the production of *Taru*, including its executive producer, director, and writers; (2) a pre-post random sample survey of 1,500 respondents each, including both listeners and non-listeners, in a sentinel research site in Begusarai District, Bihar State, India; (3) a pre-during-post, four-group, panel design quasi-experiment study to gauge the additive effects of the influence of (a) field orchestration activities such as folk performances, establishment of listening groups, and diary recordings; (b) pre-program publicity of *Taru* through posters, stickers, and flyers by the RHPs, and (c) reproductive health service delivery through the presence of a Titly Center RHP and his spouse; (4) a content analysis of a sample of listeners' letters in response to *Taru*; (5) a content analysis of the educational themes and character portrayals in the 52 episodes of *Taru*; (6) monthly collection of point-of-referral data on the sales of condoms, pills, and pregnancy dipsticks from Titly Centers in our research sites, and (7) a longitudinal design of five rapid surveys to assess the degree of audience exposure to *Taru*, conducted at two-month intervals during the broadcasts of *Taru*.

Taru's Listenership

Our five rounds of rapid exposure assessment surveys conducted in 2002 suggest that *Taru* is regularly listened to in 10 to 15 percent of all households in Begusarai District, our sentinel research site in Bihar (Table 19-1). While realizing the problems associated with estimating State-level population estimates from district-level sentinel site sample surveys, an extrapolation of these numbers suggests that *Taru* may have a listenership of between 20 to 25 million people in the four Indian States of Bihar, Madhya Pradesh, Jharkhand, and Chattisgarh, whose combined population is about 190 million people. If these listenership numbers for *Taru* hold in other Indian States (where *Taru* began broadcasting in May, 2002), the listenership of Taru in the entire Hindi-speaking region of North India, which has a total population of 625 million people, may range from 60 to 75 million people.

Community Case-Study and Field Observations

In Village Abirbur, CMS researchers and the present authors made eight rounds of visits in 2002, spending about 40 person days. Another round of visits, of roughly 20 person days, occurred in early March, 2003, soon after *Taru's* final broadcast. In September, 2002, accompanied by author Singhal, CMS researchers conducted 16 in-depth interviews and three focus group interviews (with 28 respondents) with *Taru* listeners in Abirpur, and five in-depth interviews in Village Kamtaul, including RHP Shailendra, his wife Sunita, and their daughter Vandana. These interviews were audio taped, and transcribed from Hindi into English. Our team members also investigated examples of individual and social change reported by villagers in Kamtaul, Madhopur, and Chandrahatti, spending a total of 10 person days in these sites in 2002. Various techniques of data collection were employed including participant-observation, note-taking, and photo and video documentation.

Overall Impact of *Taru*

Our study of *Taru* in Village Abirpur suggested that an entertainment-education program can spark the process of social change by drawing listeners' attention to socially desirable behaviors (Papa et. al, 2000). When listeners develop parasocial relationships with the characters of an E-E program, they may be motivated to consider changes in their own behavior. E-E programs can stimulate peer conversations among listeners, which can create opportunities for collective efficacy to emerge as people consider new patterns of thought and behavior. However, existing power structures resist the process of social change, and people's own thinking is fraught with paradoxes and contradictions as they "negotiate" their actions with their intentions. There was evidence for all these processes in the villages of Bihar, where our present investigation of *Taru* was based.

Conclusions

The *Taru* Project is intended to improve access to health services provided by rural medical practitioners in remote areas of Bihar State and to empower radio listeners in small listening groups. Our results suggest that when people organize themselves around a common purpose (in this instance, listening to a radio soap opera), the interactions help stimulate reflection, debate, and action, which may not occur for an individual listener. When individuals organize in small groups to take charge of their lives, they shift community norms, which may make the social change more sustainable.

We learned that E-E programs can spark processes of individual and social change through the formation of parasocial relationships between audience members and media characters (Horton & Wohl, 1956). Audience members consider changes in their own behavior based on what has worked or not worked for media characters. E-E programs can also initiate a process of social learning as audience members talk among themselves and consider behavior change at the individual and collective level. Some of this social learning may inspire collective action as audience members work together to improve community life (as illustrated by the newly-established open-air school in Village Abirpur).

However, individual and social change is rarely a simple, linear process. Audience members may encounter powerful forces of resistance as they attempt to change power dynamics in a community. In addition, attempts to change behavior are often fraught with paradoxes and contradictions that point to the difficulty of altering entrenched actions within complex communities. Despite these difficulties, our findings suggest that synergistic possibilities for social action emerge when entertainment-education broadcasts are integrated with community-based group listening and locally available health care services.

Assessment Dimension	Rapid Survey 1* April, 2002 (N=369)	Rapid Survey 2 June, 2002 (N=457)	Rapid Survey 3 Sept., 2002 (N=521)	Rapid Survey 4 Nov., 2002 (N=371)
Percent of *Taru* Listeners in Surveyed Households	15%	10%	12%	13%
Listeners' Perceptions of How Similar *Taru*'s Characters Are to Them	30%	48%	37%	45%
Listeners' Intentions to Change Their Behaviors as a Result of Listening to *Taru*	61%	80%	50%	83%

* Broadcasts of *Taru* began in late-February, 2002, and ended in February 2003. The rapid surveys were conducted regularly at two-month intervals.

These set of data and argument from Arvind Singhal provide important direction for entertainment-education work in Africa. They have both programmation and research implications.

Peter Vaughan made a presentation on *Using Research to Sustain Entertainment and Education Programmes*, in which he said that Entertainment-education (EE) interventions for health promotion are intended to change individual-level behaviors as part of a broader social development agenda. Because behavior change is normally a slow process, EE interventions are part of a long-term strategy that must be sustained over time, often for several years or even longer. There are three elements of sustainability with respect to EE interventions. The first element is to sustain audience interest and attention to the program. The second element is to sustain the creative team commitment and energy to the EE methodology for the duration of the intervention. Monitoring research can be used to assess both the audience attention and creative team adherence to the EE methodology elements. The third element is to sustain funding for the program. The purpose of this paper is to explore the use of *effects* research to answer important questions about intervention impact(s) on audience members' behaviors, and thereby helps to maintain donor agency commitment to the program. A long-running radio EE intervention in Tanzania is used as a case study.

Well-designed effects research is central to answering questions about program efficacy in achieving the social, health and development goals of donor agencies. There are three main questions that effects research on EE programs must answer. First, how many people listened to or watched the program? Second, over the course of broadcast, how much did the audience members change with respect to the knowledge, attitudes and particularly behaviors relevant to the donor agencies goals? Third, how much of that change is attributable to the EE intervention?

According to Vaughan, the major challenges to effects research are (1) cost, as nationally-representative survey samples are very expensive, and (2) attribution of causation to the intervention for any measured change in KAP variables. The two main strategies to overcome these challenges are (a) to partner with other surveys (for example the Demographic and Health surveys) and (b) to incorporate some sort of experimental design into the effects research.

The panelist then went on to describe the radio soap opera, *Twende na Wakati*!

Background on *Twende na Wakati* in Tanzania

"In 1992, 33 percent of Tanzanian households owned a radio and 46 percent listened to radio at least weekly, whereas only half of one percent of households owned a television set and only 3 percent watched television (Ngallaba and others, 1993). Radio Tanzania (RTD) was the primary radio signal that could be heard in many areas of the nation (POFLEP, 1994). *Twende na Wakati* ("Let's Go With the Times") was produced and broadcast by RTD in collaboration with the Ministry of Health (MOH), with technical support by Population Communications International (PCI), an NGO based in New York, and with funding from the UNFPA.

Extensive formative research for the radio soap opera was conducted in late 1992 by POFLEP (1994) (Population Family Life Education Programme), a Tanzanian research and educational center.[9] The formative research was used to develop a grid containing 57 health, economic and socio-cultural values, such as not favoring male children over female children, encouraging couples to use family planning methods, and to counter rumors such as that condom use was spreading HIV/AIDS in Tanzania (through virus in the condom lubricant). This "values grid" formed the basis for the soap opera's characters and storyline.

Three character types were featured in *TNW* to provide role models of alternative behaviors and their consequences. *Positive characters* embody the values endorsed by the values grid and were rewarded for their positive behaviors in the storyline. Fundi Mitindo and his wife Mama Waridi were two such positive role models for spousal communication, joint decision-making, and family planning adoption and were rewarded by becoming economically successful. *Negative characters* embody the negative values that the radio program intends to change, and were punished in the storyline. Mkwaju, the major negative role-model, was a promiscuous truck driver who was alcoholic, stole to support his many girlfriends and lost his job, his wife, and ultimately his life when he contracted HIV/AIDS. *Transitional characters* are initially torn by the choice between positive and negative values, but whose attitudes and behaviors evolve during the soap opera so that they eventually adopt the positive educational values and are rewarded. Tunu, Mkwaju's wife, is a transitional character, who after years of abuse by Mkwaju, first adopts family planning and later separates from Mkwaju and makes a positive life for herself and her family, thereby modeling the development of self-efficacious behavior.

An epilogue, 30 seconds or less in length, summarized the major educational issues in each radio episode, and discussed their implications for listeners. The *TNW* epilogues showed how each episode related to the daily lives of the audience individuals and promoted discussion by posing rhetorical questions.

Beginning in July 1993, Radio Tanzania broadcast *TNW* in Swahili, twice weekly during early prime-time (at 6:30 pm) for 30 minutes. The radio station at Dodoma broadcast locally produced programs at this hour, and this region served as the comparison area in our quasi-field experiment (Figure 1). The Dodoma area received all other elements of the national family planning program, including several other radio programs.

Effects research undertaken for *Twende na Wakati*

The impact of *TNW* was assessed using several independent methods. First, a study by scholars at the University of New Mexico (Rogers and others, 1999; Vaughan and others, 2000; Vaughan and Rogers, 2000) utilized (1) annual surveys of about 3,000 respondents in the comparison and treatment areas, (2) monthly clinic attendance data at 43 governmental family planning clinics in the treatment area and at 27 clinics in the comparison area from 1990 to 1996, (3) a 20 percent sample of new clients at the same clinics were asked about their source of referral, (4) condom distribution to the treatment and comparison areas by the National AIDS Control Program (NACP) from 1990 to 1997, and (5) several other qualitative methods. Second, four Demographic and Health Surveys (the 1991/92 Demographic and Health Survey (Ngallaba and others, 1993), the 1994 Knowledge, Attitudes, and Practices Survey (Weinstein and others, 1995), the 1996 Demographic and Health Survey (Bureau of Statistics and Macro International, 1997), and the 1999 Reproductive and Child Health Survey (National Bureau of Statistics and Macro International, 2000) were analyzed by Vaughan (2003) for any effects of the radio soap opera on family planning adoption.

Results

Between 1960 and 1999, the population size of Tanzania more than tripled from 10.2 million to 34.3 million (Figure 2). However, the inflection point of the growth curve was also reached in the 1990s, indicating a slowing in the rate of population growth, and the UN medium projection for the next 50 years is that the population will about double in size to 70 million people by 2050. Figure 2 indicates that after a long period of stasis, the total fertility rate (TFR) in Tanzania began to decline from about 6.8 in 1980, and then declined rapidly in the 1990s before stabilizing at about 5.6 in 1994. The steepest point of the decline in TFR corresponds to the beginning of broadcasting of *TNW*, but this correlation does not necessarily imply that *TNW* was the cause of the decline in TFR.

Listenership to *TNW* in the comparison area was very low in 1995 (2 percent) but there was marked regional variation in the listenership with much higher listenership in several coastal regions and much lower listenership in several western regions. This provides for a "natural experiment" in which one would hypothesize that one should see greater change in those regions where listenership was higher. The DHS surveys measured a high national listenership to *TNW* in 1996 of 40 percent for men and 23 percent for women, and in 1999 this increased to 51 percent for men and 31 percent for women.

Vaughan and Rogers (2000) developed a six-stage model of behavior change for family planning adoption. Using the four DHS surveys, respondents were assigned to (1) the Maintenance stage if they were currently using a modern family planning method, (2) the Action stage if they had ever used a modern family planning method and did not belong to a higher stage, (3) the Validation stage if they had talked about family planning with their partner at least once and did not belong to a higher stage, (4) the Preparation stage if they intended to use a family planning method in the future, approved of the use of family planning methods, and did not belong to a higher stage, (5) the Contemplation stage if they knew of at least one modern family planning method and did not belong to a higher stage, and (6) the Pre-contemplation stage if they knew of no modern family planning methods and did not belong to a higher stage.

For both men and women there is a statically significant increase in average stage score in the treatment area from 1991/92 (pre-broadcast) to 1994 (post-broadcast in the treatment area, pre-broadcast in the comparison area). Women increased by an average of 0.6 stages and men increased by an average of 1.2 stages during this period (Vaughan, 2003). By contrast in the comparison area, the average stage score for women increased by only 0.1, and for men by 0.2, but neither increase was statistically significant. There is a significant increase for women for the period 1991/92 to 1996 (increase of 0.3 stages, ANOVA, p<. 01) and for men for the period 1991/92 to 1999 (increase of 0.7 stages, ANOVA, p< .001) (broadcasts of TNW began in the comparison area in 1995). It is more difficult to show statistical significance in the comparison area because there were smaller sample sizes there (N = 225 to 635 for women; N = 93 to 175 for men).

The results of regional-level linear regression analyses (Vaughan, 2003), included the effects of (1) being in the treatment or comparison area, (2) the natural experiment effect of the regional level of exposure to *TNW* or *Zinduka!* and (3) 42 other control variables. Only 7 variables were significant in the final model, with the treatment effect being the most important. Being in the treatment area accounted for an increase in approximately 0.5 stages, while each 10-percentage point increase in regional listenership increased the model stage by about 0.1 stages. The R^2 value for this regression was 0.77, or this model explains more than three-fourths of the variation in regional change in model stage.

We analysed the mean number of new and continuing family planning adopters at 43 MOH clinics in the treatment area and at 27 clinics in the comparison area from January 1990 through December 1996. The trend lines for the treatment and comparison areas increased at approximately the same rate during the pre-broadcast period from January 1990 to June 1993. The treatment slope is 0.7 (SE = .05) and the comparison area slope is 0.5 (SE = .30); the 95 percent confidence limits for the two trend lines almost always overlap during this pre-intervention period.

From July 1993 through September 1995, when the radio soap opera was broadcast in the treatment area only, the slope in the treatment area increases to 1.6 (SE = .21), while the slope in the comparison area increases only slightly, to 0.6 (SE = .11). During this field experimental period, the 95 percent confidence bars do not overlap for most months. After September 1995, the trend line in the treatment area plateaus, while the slope in the former comparison area increases to 1.2 (SE = .45), and the 95 percent confidence bars mostly overlap, as the rate of adoption in the former comparison area catches up with the treatment area. This pattern supports the hypothesis that *TNW* stimulated an increase in the rate of family planning adoption when it was broadcast first in the treatment area and later in the comparison area after 1995.

From 1994 to 1998, 25 percent (N = 3,739) of the new family planning adopters at 49 Ministry of Health clinics in the treatment area reported in answer to an unaided recall question that their main source/channel of referral in adopting family planning was *TNW* (or *TNW* plus another information source).

Data from the UNM study (Vaughan and others, 2000), shows that AIDS was nearly universally known in Tanzania by 1993. However, respondents suffered both from a lack of information about how AIDS is transmitted and how to protect oneself from the disease, and from misinformation. The average score on an AIDS knowledge scale was 10.0 in the treatment area and 10.9 in the comparison area in 1993 (out of a maximum of 14). During the two year period of 1993 to 1995, the AIDS knowledge score increased by 0.7 points in the treatment area and declined by 0.5 points in the comparison area, due in part to the increased belief that condoms spread the HIV virus. From 1995 to 1997, knowledge leveled off in the treatment area, but increased by 0.3 points in the comparison area after broadcasts of *TNW* began there.

We did an analysis of data on whether respondents felt that they were personally at risk of contracting HIV/AIDS. In the treatment area, this variable increased during both time periods, but it declined in the comparison area during the first time period (before broadcast of *TNW* in that area) and then increased dramatically[1] (21 percentage points) once broadcasts of *TNW* began there. These data are important because many people believe that individuals will only change their behavior once they understand that they are personally at risk of contracting the disease.

The most important behavior change that we were able to measure was a change in the number of sexual partners that both men and women claimed to have had in the previous year. There was a secular downward trend in this variable of about 0.3 partners for men and 0.5 partners for women, but the decline was greater in the treatment area than it was in the comparison area.

We were also able to document an increased demand for condoms, that occurred first in the treatment area and then in the comparison area after 1995. The large fluctuations in the condom data are due to logistical problems encountered in the importation of condoms, especially in 1995.

Discussion and Conclusions

"I pray to the radio management to extend the program for at least another three years. During the new phase I would request that Mkwaju's behavior be changed to a positive role model as he has suffered a lot and let another character assume the negative role."

Male letter-writer to TNW, Dar Es Salaam. Tanzania.

As data presented here and in Vaughan (2003) demonstrate, important information about effects of EE interventions can be obtained at relatively low cost by collaborating with other organizations, such as the Demographic and Health Surveys, to obtain high-quality and nationally representative data. While normally only a relatively few questions can be inserted into these questionnaires, the surveys are often designed to ask about important knowledge, attitudes and behaviors relevant to many health promotions campaigns. Once questions about the EE intervention are inserted into the survey instrument, statistical analyses can be conducted to explore relationships between the (1) exposure variables, (2) other independent variables, such as socio-economic variables, and (2) important health dependent variables. Because surveys are repeated in many countries at relatively short intervals, they can be used to measure change over periods of 3 to 5 years.

The most rigorous manner to demonstrate a causal relationship is through the creation of a control area which does not receive the EE intervention but is monitored, at about the same level of intensity, as a treatment area. However, the deliberate withholding of potentially live-saving information from a region poses serious ethical ramifications now that the potential effects of EE interventions has been demonstrated (e.g.

Culture, Entertainment and Health Promotion

Vaughan and others, 1999). These ethical concerns are ameliorated by the use of "natural" rather than deliberate experiments, which are created by regional or geographical variation in exposure to the EE intervention. While these natural experiments do not carry the statistical rigor of true experiments, the do allow the attribution of causation provided the assumption that exposure levels to the EE intervention are independent of other factors related to the behavior change of study. This may be reasonable in many circumstances, but not all. For example, low listenership to *TNW* in some areas of Tanzania may have been due to poor transmission in those areas from old/ineffective transmitters, but this poor communication development may also co-vary with the regional ability to provide family planning services, which may be the real reason for lack of family planning behavior change observed in those areas. This concern of a regional variation in levels of development that cuts across development sectors (e.g., communications and health) can cause spurious correlations between measured level of exposure to and EE intervention and change in a health behavior. True experimental designs are the only way to surmount this concern.

Twende na Wakati has been financially supported by the UNFPA for ten years, enabling it to remain "on air" much longer than most EE programs. During this time, the Ministry of Health, and other Tanzanian Ministries have broadened its agenda from the original Family planning and HIV/AIDS prevention objectives, to incorporate other development initiatives. This financial and institutional support is most likely attributable to the clear demonstration of the impact of *TNW* in furthering the social and health development goals of the UNFPA and the Tanzanian government."

The radio soap opera, *Twende na Wakati* has become a national institution and quite often government and partners call on the producer to incorporate priority issues. After the 2004 Bangkok Conference the theme of HIV/AIDS was integrated into the storyline more systematically and deliberately. The values matrix was adjusted to reflect the role of family in prevention, care and support.

Things to ponder about:

- Listener clubs create a medium of continuous media. The broadcasting of the programme in India was limited to 20 villages and quality control as an orchestrator is not easy. It is not easy to maintain listener groups and the best listening group that is intact is the family. This has worked for the Indian context. The listener groups in India are registered and the incentive is to be recognized on air.

- If as a producer you have listener groups set to discuss specific issues, then you are not telling the story but trying to deal with issues in that particular society. How then do you pass the idea that people are part of the programme? Listeners need to be given an issue and then let them decide whether they want to engage or not. However if a programme is entertaining, listeners will find it interesting and stay on.

- In *Ushikwapo*, there are listeners clubs modelled within the drama. This has prompted the formation of about 130 clubs that have resulted spontaneously. These groups are now connected through greeting cards that are read on air during the programmes. This is indicative of the influence outside the drama. How can such groups be sustained?

- The relationship between research and art is critical. There is a notion that if there is feeling and passion, then research is irrational. But passion can be used to manipulate. There are different methods encumbered in philosophies. In research, we try to have a multi method approach. In terms of design, that is, formative research, it is important for each of the philosophies to play a part. In terms of methodology, it takes a special creative talent to create a soap opera.

XI

Writing and Producing Issue Based Entertainment Programs

Art has been, is, and will always be necessary. Among other things art creates in human beings a sense of 'fullness'; wholeness. We are uncomfortable with being lone individuals; unconnected by phenomena beyond ourselves. Art provides the linkages and creates a world that seems to make sense to us by tying the pieces of apparently disparate phenomena. We resist, by experiencing art, the confines of our own lives, the transient limitations of our individuality. The I is not enough and we long to embrace the world around us. We seek to make individuality *social* by bringing into our lives those 'others' that will enrich the 'self' Art becomes our indispensable and inalienable tool for the bridging of the individual with the whole. In its associativeness, art helps us share thoughts and experiences and makes us better human beings.

Artists seize and transform experiences and memory into a form that they enjoy and apprehend. The experiences, however, are not presented in their raw form but are mediated and constructed anew. The construction makes art captive and hold its audience and this temporary captivity is entertaining because it is pleasurable.

A socially relevant art seeks to grip the audience and goes further: it appeals to reason, not through passive identification, but rather by an appeal to cognition which demands decision and action. The type of art I am talking about targets the critical consciousness and ignites action – a responsible consciousness.

Human beings are story tellers (homo narans) and they learn best through stories and experiences. In EE programs, it is possible to integrate knowledge and emotion into the programs so that audience members increase what they know, change their attitudes and adopt certain behaviour. This is done through effective characterization, dexterity in nesting of stories and powerful artistic tools (metaphor, simile, symbolism) and language use.

Many EE programs now include markers in their design. Markers are distinctive elements of a message that are identifiable by audience members. In the St. Lucia radio soap opera Apwe Plezi the condom was referred to as a **'catapult'** and in the Kenyan soap it was called **'puto'**. Characters could be named creatively such as 'Mkwaju' in the Tanzanian soap 'Twende na Wakati'. Mkwaju became a common part of popular discourse in Tanzania. In addition, writers could model new, culturally appropriate realities which are replicated in the real world (such as collective show of disapproval by honking of cars or banging of pots and pans).

The liberative aspects of art – through its ability to help in the transformation of reality – results from its unique ability to move us from a state of fragmentation to a state of wholeness; of integration.

But how do the writers and producers of EE programs view the matters? The summit invited panelists to share their experiences.

(The panel consisted of Martha Swai of Radio Tanzania, Tanzania-Dar Es Salaam, Tanzania; King Dube/Nicola Harford of Center 4 , Zimbabwe and Binyavanga Wainaina, editor of the *Kwani?* electronic journal, Kenya. The session was chaired by Ashina Kibibi, a producer an artist form Kenya. The panelists walked the participants through the various methodologies that they use to produce E-E programs).

Following on comments made by Peter Vaughan, Martha Swai made a presentation on *Producing an Issue Based Soap Opera: The Case of Twende na Wakati*. She introduced the session by pointing out that communication is a very vital process underlying changes in knowledge. Therefore, the development of messages and materials that can increase knowledge, change of attitudes and encourage behavior change go hand in hand with good presentation of the said message.

The *Twende Na Wakati* soap opera started in 1993 to address the issues of family planning; maternal mortality and women empowerment; harmful traditional practices; STIs and HIV/AIDS.

The program was developed in collaboration with Population Communications International and thus follows the PCI methodology, which constitutes research, the use of values grids, script development, technical review and production. Kimani Njogu and Tom Kazungu provided the gist of the technical support to the artists.

Following the PCI methodology a baseline research was conducted to identify gaps and issues; to obtain an accurate picture of local, cultural, economic and health circumstances and to identify local attitudes and practices on such issues as reproductive health issues, family size, gender roles, STIs and HIV/AIDS.

The major issues identified that needed to be highlighted in *Twende Na Wakati* were fertility and family planning; HIV/AIDS; girl child education; harmful traditional practices including FGC/M and gender equity and equality. Thus, these issues were incorporated into the Moral Framework, which served as a framework for the development and writing of stories. For instance, in 2002 stories focused on fertility issues and values; family planning issues; maternal and child health issues; sexually transmitted infections and HIV/AIDS; gender equity and equality issues and social cultural issues, among others.

Script Development

Twende na Wakati has five scriptwriters Salim Nkamba, Michael Kadinde, Mayasa Jengo, Makoye and Mbena who work together to develop the scripts from which the radio programs are produced. The major planning is done annually where major themes for the year are identified. Consequently, the holding of weekly meetings to plan together and discuss issues, characters and the story line are discussed is done throughout the year.

Martha Swai went on to say that the language used is guided by the story and has to be appealing to the specific audiences. A Technical Review Committee goes through the scripts to ensure correctness of technical information.

Recording Rehearsals
Recording is done in the Radio Tanzania studios after rehearsals. There is an effort to ensure that the message is educative and interesting. The mood of presentation – angry, sad or happy - adds to the weight of the script.

Feedback

"Feedback is important for the scriptwriters. Feedback helps the program producers and scriptwriters to give appropriate messages for their audiences. Feedback is received through audience letters and field monitoring visits. Feedback also enables the team to identify areas which need improvement; it sheds light on the type of audience, the appropriateness of language use and the effectiveness of the messages relayed. Creativeness and flexibility are very important in the presentation of the message for social change," she said.

Martha Swai has been the producer of *Twende na Wakati* for many years. She works extremely closely with her team, seven days a week to ensure the success of this phenomenal intervention. Unfortunately, the program is dependent on UNFPA. Due to the poor state of the Tanzania economy, advertisers do not undertake to support the program. Most advertisers target the middle class but our entertainment-programs mainly target the poor and marginalized who do not have money to shop aggressively. This is the problem.

King Dube and Nicola Harford made a presentation on *The MARCH Strategy*, a program on behavior change communication strategies for HIV/AIDS prevention and mitigation that rolls out to Zimbabwe, Botswana and Ethiopia.

Harford went on to talk about role modeling and reinforcement to combat HIV/AIDS and behavioral change achieved through *Mopani Junction*: a long-running (two year) radio serial drama, and the reinforcement of the modeled behavior change achieved through community level activities and interpersonal communication.

Entertainment-Education

She explained why her organization prefers to use radio serial drama. This is because based on behavior change theory – social learning theory that uses role models – people learn from observing others. They provide alternative narratives that emphasize entertainment. However, change occurs at a realistic pace as people move through stages of change.

Behavioral Objectives

Through the years the organizational goals for the program has been to increase the proportion of young adults aged 15-29 years who delay initiation of sexual intercourse; practice safe sex (abstinence, mutual monogamy, correct and consistent use of condoms); learn their HIV status and live with the results (stay negative or if positive, live positively; if pregnant enroll on PMTCT program) and support the infected and affected.

On the conceptual framework for *MARCH*, the objective of the formative research is to obtain information needed to develop storylines that reflect the reality of young adults' experiences, and design the reinforcement activities. After research, data summary grids are developed.

Data lists were divided into barriers and facilitators and grouped into categories. Barriers and facilitators relate to access to care; alcohol and substance abuse; cultural shift and westernization; gender issues, roles and problems; inter-generational issues; materialism/economic pressure; relationships among peers; HIV/AIDS and sexual knowledge and practices and stigma.

The *Pathways to Change* tools utilize board Game (using the data summary grids). Behavior Change Charts used include speech acts; pathways to Change Game; building familiarity with research data; learning key behavior change concepts; identifying barriers and facilitators to behavior change in reference to a specific character (e.g. male, female, young, old married, unmarried) living in a specific setting (rural, urban). It also includes the distribution events in a transitional character's "behavior change trajectory" over a period of time and observing how a series of behavior change events look in terms of the "stages of change" (and revise, if necessary) and keeping track of transitional characters' behavior change trajectories.

Mopani Junction has a format of implementation: In the two years the program has been aired in three language versions - Shona, Ndebele and English for 30 minutes per episode. Each scene is three minutes and eight scenes per episode. Music is included in the episodes. Narration and previews and Vox Pops / epilogues / competitions are included.

The background is about Josh, a 19-year-old school-leaver, raised by a single mother, who does not know his father, and wants to pursue a career in music. The *barriers* he faces are peer pressure, alcohol and an economic need. However, the facilitators for Josh are long-term goals, knowledge of risk.

The other story is on voluntary counseling and testing (VCT) and Living positively. A 26-year-old rural woman with abusive husband, Mishek, and daughters Ruth and Mutsa. The *barriers* in this story are gender relations; lack of education and information; low self-efficacy, fear of stigma. *Facilitators* are a social support and an income-generating scheme.

Production Cycle:
This involves script development; concept/storyline; review by Technical Advisory Committee; step outline and dialogue writing production includes rehearsals and recording and post-production activities."

The experience brought to the Summit by *Mopani Junction* shows that the use of popular artistic creations when well designed can and do make a difference.

Ashina Kibibi is well known for the production of Tausi, a Kenyan TV serial. She made a presentation on: *Writing and Producing Issue-Based Entertainment Programs.*

According to Kibibi "an issue as a subject of significant concern to the society." The beginning point for "issue" based entertainment programme has therefore to be the subject one decides to address. The writer has to identify a subject in the society which is important and exciting.

"The type of issue to be addressed will be determined by various factors. It could depend on the society itself (its cultures, demography, traditions) or it could be determined by the circumstances that are prevailing in the society (i.e. high rates of HIV/AIDS infections, international terrorism).

In identifying the issue to be addressed, the writer must ask the following:

- Is the subject a matter of significant concern to the society? Is it serious enough to warrant the effort you are about to put into it?

- Is the issue relevant? Are you about to blow a non – issue out of proportion?

- Do you have a proper perspective on the issue? Do you appreciate the issue and its many perspectives and have you chosen the proper one? i.e. when addressing the issue of early marriages, are you addressing the uprooting of young girls from school or lack of romantic freedom for young girls? Is your perspective the same as that of the society at large? If not, is your perspective relevant to the concerns of the society at large?

- Is the issue short – term or long – term? Is it a short – term issue with the long – term effects like for instance, a national election, or is it a continuous long – term issue like tribalism or HIV/AIDS?

This understanding is relevant in deciding how to deal with the issue from an artistic approach."

The next thing to have in mind according to Kibibi is the purpose of the production. The fundamental purpose of the issue-based programme is to inform, generate debate and make the viewer address the issue by action. It differs from a normal entertainment programme in this respect. It is possible to fully entertain the viewers and at the same time address the issue. One must therefore go beyond entertainment to speak to the intellect of the viewer and therefore get a chance to address an issue. The first point is to decide on the nature of the programme to be produced. Is it political, social, economic? Each has its distinct characteristic and must be addressed from a different artistic approach. For instance, a political issue is good material for satire, traditional conflicts are good material for comedies and health issues are best addressed through tragedy.

Apart from understanding the issue, one must also properly understand the society of viewers. What are their values, religion, and the demography? Understanding the society helps in determining the style of the writer, the words you use, the balancing between dialogues an action. For instance, a religious society has to be approached with polite literature. A Young viewer society prefers more Drama than dialogue. A society of educated people may want some philosophical approach in the script. These decisions should be made after proper understanding of the society itself.

She informed participants that when she wrote the TV serial TAUSI, she wrote an episode (No 27) where a Muslim girl performed an abortion and a Muslim woman went to consult a witchdoctor. "I wanted to deal with the hypocrisy of human nature and how humans are punished for this hypocrisy. However, I wrote the issue over several episodes, the punishment coming to episode 35. The uproar that came from the episode 27 almost derailed the entire programme. I learnt that suspense is not an effective tool in religious matters and that I should have dealt with the hypocrisy and the punishment in the same episode. The same approach would however have worked on another issue that did not touch on religion. This understanding is also necessary when dealing with production. When producing, one goes through auditioning and casting, costumes, locations, shooting and editing. Let us see how an overall knowledge of the issue and the society affects one' approach in production."

Auditioning and Casting

The actor that one chooses must portray the character effectively. Usually social stereotypes determine the nature of the character. For instance, in *TAUSI,* the lead role was a rich and strict Muslim man. "We had to cast a tall, well-built Man with a likable character. Our thinking was that among our viewers, the height and built would be viewed as a sense of authority that was natural whereas similar strictness form a short character would be viewed as cruel.

We would also have to cast a prostitute who would not be hated by the viewers and who would generate concern and debate. We cast a beautiful plump lady with a motherly aura. The viewers looked at her as a Lady who would be a good wife if she agreed to settle down. Viewer discussed her character and suggested what she would do with her life. We felt that a slim prostitute would have been taken by viewers as irredeemable and would not generate any interest in her favor. Size in women is seen as sign of contentment. Viewers do not psychologically accept a lean cut Man as prosperous."

Casting is important because a wrongly cast character will find it difficult to convince the viewer. They will not embody the character being represented. The result is that the message on the issue is lost. Viewers lose interest and feel the actor is cheating them. "In *TAUSI*, we changed the main male character by the name *Mjuba* and the changes did not convince the viewers who thought the new actor was not as talented or physically striking. We lost many viewers in both Kenya and Tanzania as a result."

Costumes

Costume is important in bringing out the realism in a character. It is important in visually enhancing the role. If the programme is to deliver the message or excite debate, it must ensure that the viewers accept its characters. And a character wearing the wrong outfit will confuse the viewer.

Locations

In most local productions, there is little attention to locations. Most programmes are based on one scene and the drama revolves around this scene. Locations are important because they break monotony of the programme, enhance the reality of the character the reality of the drama.

Shooting , Scoring & Editing

A good story can be lost in the shooting and editing stages. Shooting determines what the viewer finally sees. Good acting, good costume and good choice of locations are useless if the intended effect is not recorded.

The types of shots used bring out a different aspect of drama or dialogue. One must therefore have in mind what the message is and what method of delivery has been chosen. The use of music and sound effects will be added advantage. Music can be used in either enhancing the emotions or attracting the viewers. The late Fundi Konde modeled the title TAUSI on the song TAUSI. That title and the use of the song in the play attracted a lot of viewers to the series. A part from holding the attention of those who are watching, music can win you more viewers giving you a chance to spread your message further.

In choosing music, we must understand the society. The choice of music must relate to the viewers. A good song for one society is not good for another". With those remarks, Kibibi concluded her reflections.

Things to ponder about:

- The process of working on *Mopani Junction* felt like the matrix was being reloaded. There is something about theory in a place where people have been subjected to state media. The onus is on the institutions to come up with ways of approaching creative artists.

- Writing scripts and incorporating writers has not been easy. Writing has its own dynamics but it is important that writers get paid well and their integrity respected. We need to promote free expression.

- This meeting is a very good forum since we have writers, donors and artists sitting in one room. We are getting into a stage where we are experiencing problems with writers and artists due to remuneration. We should pay them better so that we have improved productions.

- The question of what is the African story is always an issue. As a writer, one is forced to draw on what is a universal story. However, it is important that each story must have its own heartbeat and nurture it up to its life. Writers also need to be part of the research teams for productions.

XII

Sustainability: A Possibility or a Mirage?

An ongoing challenge for EE programs is sustainability. How will the program continue once donors pull out? Most stakeholders would like programs to continue once funds are unavailable. But this is not always the case. Governments, commercial sponsorships, NGOs and CBOs can play an important role in ensuring that there is continuity. How are EE programs coping? We posed this question to the Summit participants.

(The panelists were David Campbell of Mediae, Kenya; Yvonne Adhiambo of the Zanzibar International Film Festival (ZIFF), Zanzibar and Elizabeth Mwaila of The German Technical Cooperation (GTZ), Kenya. The session was chaired by Tom Kazungu of Apex Productions).

David Campbell began by pointing out that to ensure sustainability, it is important to undertake research to find out the audience' needs, in terms of content and listenership. This enables the production of good programs that meet the needs of the audience. If research reveals high audience ratings and measurable changes, then there will be interest in sponsorship. He continued by saying that development partners/donors for any radio serial dramas could include the target audiences - e.g. rural / poor (conflict communities) and age/socio economic groups. Some of the issues that the serial drama by MEDIAE highlights and tackles include issues of gender.

"To establish if the messages are relevant to the target groups it is very important for each of our soaps to be evaluated and monitored. For such an end we come up with indicators such as measures of change in KAPB - Does it work? We establish the numbers of program listeners. We also try to meet the predetermined donor objectives/audiences needs. Message content, quantity and time to get information over is important for any serial drama. Thus, accessibility to recommendations so change can take place is inherent.

However, it is also important to note that different clients have different needs and different source of support. Our main challenge as programmers for social change come across is that the media in Kenya and the world over is very commercialised making it very expensive for us to run our programs in the most competitive stations. This is so because we have to pay for the airtime instead of letting the advertiser handle it. By doing so they are paid the 18% placement fee, they are less likely to complain (Loss of production fee) and new ads would appear more regularly. The duty of the program producers would be would to be on the look out for new fads and offer advertising agencies placement in their programs. They would also be in a position to argue the social responsibility links etc with the radio stations to make airtime less expansive and affordable by sharing it out with the many partners.

Since different clients have different needs and support it is important for us to identify development partners/donors to pay for content - for production, research, development. Different collaborates, different strands. Working with these varied kinds of people/ collaborators in our endeavours to give them access to our drama content, field work/links and involving them in develop research with them - baseline and follow up, quarterly reporting to someone who cares! Discussing other media links would start renewal processes early and contracts possible. This involvement ensures that program sustainability does not solely depend on donor aid but on other creative innovations".

He gave a case of how the Mediae's radio serial drama *Tembea Na Majira* does it:

Airtime
The soap drama is 15 minutes long. It is aired on Thursdays at 8.15 pm and is repeated on Sundays at 8.15 pm. It also constitutes a Magazine programme. On a larger picture, the drama totals 45 minutes of radio time weekly. Airtime costs approximately US $1000 per 15 minutes. Weekly costs about US $3,000 and the annual cost is approximately US $156,000. On the other hand, it costs the advertising agency about 18% of the whole airtime cost. That is in this case US $28,080. Ordinarily the advertisers get reductions.

Production costs:

- Programme production per episode is approximately US $72,000. The soap costs US $600 while the magazine costs US $400. Totalling to about US $1,000 per week and an equivalent of US $52,000 per year

- Research costs about US $20,000 per year.

To help meet these costs Mediae have three sponsors who donate about US $24,000. This is significant in view of audience numbers (about six million).

Issues/ Radio

It is important for social change soaps to tackle issues so as to ensure that airtime gives added value to client base. They commissioned independent researchers who support this information and donor demands. Keeping costs down so as to make sure donor costs are low is one way that can be used to make possible longer term contracts and to attract different levels of partners to get on board. Others can use limited funding that is available.

Issues /TV

In Kenya today there a few limiting challenges to these efforts that include:

- Much higher local costs for production
    - Between $5,000 to $100,000 per one hour programme
- Large English speaking audience /Cheap imports
    - $500 for 10 year old *Bold and Beautiful;*
    - Need to compete with these;
    - Limited advertising budgets allows donor/message dominance in the market.

David Campbell suggests that entertainment education programs can be self sustaining but continuous research in order to bring on board advertisers is vital. Advertisers want numbers. But as stated earlier, many of them target clients who can buy. Many people in Africa survive on less than a dollar a day and are not of value to the profit driven economic system. In addition, globalization is weakening creativity in Africa through cheap imports.

Margaret Mwaila presented her piece on *HIV/AIDS at the Workplace*. She began by stressing the fact that in Kenya today 10% of the population is infected by HIV, the virus that causes AIDS (Surveillance 2002). The most affected age groups are 19 – 49years and 50% of infections occur in youth below 25 years. 30-40% infections are vertical – MTCT while 864 AIDS-related deaths occur daily (MoH, 2003). There are over one million orphans due to HIV/AIDS. Women are twice likely to be infected compared to men. But why do we need to respond to HIV/AIDS at the workplace? This is because we are all at risk– companies as well as individuals.

Mwaila said; "As businesses, we need to produce quality products and services. To stay in the market we aim at efficiency and cost-effectiveness. We must care for our communities – they are our business!"

GTZ's activities in HIV/AIDS started in 90s among the rural-based and agricultural programs. Together with the Rural Health Program (RHP) and support from the headquarters, HIV/AIDS project initiative was put in place in 1998. The program adopted the use of the Peer Educator Program (volunteer FPs) and training. It has a mandate to spend 3% of total government funding to HIV/AIDS.

The goals include reduction in HIV prevalence among staff and contact communities. Support mechanisms are available and accessible to all staff and contact communities. The program attains and sustains behavior change by equipping all staff and contact communities with continuous (behavior Change Education) BCE/Information.

GTZ's Workplace Policy addresses subtle issues in the workplace policy which include prevention, care and support; non-discrimination and de-stigmatization of infected and affected; HIV testing not a condition for employment. Through advocacy, employees are advised to seek VCT services; confidentiality is maintained for infected staff and their families. HIV/AIDS has been mainstreamed into the core business of all GTZ-supported projects/ programs in Kenya through adoption of the multisectoral/multi-pronged approach, use of the Peer Educator approach, and setting up a staff HIV scheme to benefit infected staff and families. GTZ sensitizes staff and contact communities on STIs and HIV/AIDS, trains volunteers in PE, BCC, Advocacy and PC, develops and disseminates BCC, PMTCT and Nutrition information/materials. It also conducts condom education and distribution, setting up resource center(s), and provision of VCT advocacy. Implementation of a staff HIV scheme and networking are some of their activities. The benefits of mainstreaming HIV/AIDS have resulted in cost-saving, and efficient and effective iterventions. There is a highly sensitized staff and communities meaning better life skills (e.g. prevention using safer sex). There is an established and implementation of workplace policy.

The GTZ- Kenya staff HIV scheme and initiative has received best practice recognition and interest to replicate it e.g. from GTZ UG, SDC, Engender Health, etc.

There is also the promotion of healthcare service seeking behavior. Capacity building ensures high motivation and setting and building up the resource center(s). Another achievement has been the development, production and dissemination of BCC, PMTCT and nutrition information; including promotion of condom use. The challenges encountered include lack of strengthened surveillance and documentation at the national level, funding, volunteerism and commitment, and the fact that this new initiative is still evolving.

Sustainability is a possibility if there is political goodwill, partnerships to ensure quality and quantity in terms of resource mobilization and collective involvement of all stakeholders right from project conceptualization. Other ways would be to have low-cost initiatives e.g. mainstreaming, dialogue, use of locally available resources, innovation, on -the-job training, transparency and accountability at all levels and continuous monitoring.

It is imperative for the governments to recognize the work that is being done by the social change programmers and their contribution to society. Since many of such programs are delivered through government channels, assistance should be given by the respective governments through reduced airtime and subsidized rates to name a few. Through this support, creators and producers of E-E programs would be in a better position to afford, develop and continue their work."

Focusing on work places for AIDS intervention has value due to the ability of target audience members to continue dialogue as they work. But this calls for cooperation from managers and chief executives who might view the interventions as interfering in production. The value of a healthy labour force for productivity would need to be reiterated.

Film as a tool of social change is still in its infancy in Africa. More needs to be done here.

Yvonne Adhiambo, gave an *Overview of the Experiences of the Zanzibar International Film Festival.* She began by asking participants to imagine of a certain creature often, unfortunately, associated with the mythical Swamp thing. It has more lives than cat, a hide thicker than the oldest rhinoceros, a mind that is a cross between Einstein's and the Octopus, the forked tongue of the devil (donation in-kind) and the DNA of a chameleon. It survives in all environments but also has the power of transmogrification. It can become something else even as it is telling you it is one thing. It is NOT the TAO, nor is it connected in any way to the Return of the Messiah, though it could be if it becomes politically correct. It makes friends in high places and also low. The creature's clarion call is multi-voiced, but is best known by its morning voice-*Ngongongo*. Which is where it derives its collective name, the one we know it by, NGO.

A friend, lets us call him William. He joined the ancestors, we can paraphrase him freely. Well, William suggested: Some NGOs are born sustainable. Others achieve sustainability and still others have sustainability thrust upon them.

"Somewhere in 1996-1997, a bunch of people got together in Zanzibar and decided to dream, a common occurrence on that lovely island. Some of the dreamers were from Zanzibar. Others just lived there. And still others were shipwrecked there, also common occurrence. Well, they gathered around a table at the Head of Television's office in this land of dhows and said: let there be a fest of films that will bring together, in Zanzibar, the peoples and countries of the world in which dhows may have, should have or still ply their trade.

The dreamers gathered other dreamers around them until there were many dreamers from many countries in Zanzibar, some of who were from a very important specie of humans called 'Donors'.

In 1998, it was all made official with an official Board of Directors and an official certificate that said "NGO" written on it-but not exactly in those words-and an official authority to do all that appertains to being an NGO. The donors were also delighted and gave lots of money, enough to hold a small film festival. It was all managed from the inner office of the office of one of the dreamers who was now officially called "Board Member 'of the Zanzibar International Film Festival, and in the manner of all good NGOs, this was acronymised into ZIFF.

The next year the donors were even happier. Zanzibar is an even lovelier place in late June, early July, when the Festival, now known as the ZIFF Festival of the dhow countries unfolds. Well the donors were happy and gave even more money.

The next year the donors were delirious with a joy deeper than the previous years and ZIFF found a serious suitor who even gave more money for the festival. The film festival had meanwhile, acquired a few other limbs; a music of the festival wing, a seminar of the festival wing, a social development communications wing-called the Panoramas which allowed the donors to see the words they liked: Children, Women, Rural village. ZIFF was happy. The donors were happy.

Alas, though, the donors had not asked about IMs. IMs are institutional mechanisms. They did not ask about the 'IMs' in the place to administer the money because everyone was so happy about the great idea whose time had come. And ZIFF being an NGO did not ask what the donors did not ask and this blissful non-asking state continued until 2001-2 when suddenly--maybe it is because ZIFF had, in its zeal, sort of spent a little more than it should have spent in the festival that had grown and grown and grown, --donors got a little cross with ZIFF. Which is not to say that this were also years of serious spending cut-backs and the arrival in Zanzibar of an interesting little word 'sustainability'. Since it is an S word and it has a hissing sound, I am afraid there may have been people who thought it was a dirty word and decided to ignore it, as is the right thing to do when accosted by a dirty word.

There is a whole other story of how a bunch of dreamers and donors have been forced by each other's presence and a shared passion for a vision that they are aware cannot be allowed to die, to embrace a practical, painful, definite and determine path to institutional sustainability. The short version is this: the restructuring and re-education of the ZIFF Board and staff-enabled by the donors, the installation of management accounting systems: facilitated by the donors, and the installation of a cold-hearted accountant with a whiny voice. Also the recruitment of multi-skilled managers with exposure to corporate practice. These managers have been asked by the Board to incorporate corporate methodologies into the set up. With this type of management, another vocabulary is-maybe sadly-entering into the ZIFF realm:

1. Staff as marketers, organizational positioning, corporate partnerships, the festival brand, the organization brand and in the name of all that is holy, not donors, but institutional partners or programme investors.

2. Adaptation of corporate sustainability road markers: annual plan, strategic plans, management by objectives, departmental responsibility, profit center mentality (meaning, each section aims to sustain itself), marketing plans.

3. Identity: vision, mission, objectives, organizational, festival, products, the who we are, what do we do, what do others imagine we are, what do others want us to be/do, what survival strategy do we adopt:

4. (a) evolution (b) resistance (c) termination (e) extinction (f) Ostrich bury head in the sand and it will go away).

5. Very important, I believe: Product focus. What do we have others want? What else can we produce, with whom and how? And with a product focus a look at a product's life span and looking at distribution mechanisms beyond the borders, seeking partners beyond the present milieu. Diversification: ideas, partners, products. Consolidation: ideas, partners, products

In short, starting to look at the BUSINESS of the organization and the festival and so on.

The forced evolution of ZIFF into a corporate savvy organization is at the fist levels. But will it change the original dream? I do not know. But there have been some noticeable changes. Staff vocabularies now include time lines, six month plans, corporate partnerships, product growth feedback and departmental co-coordinators talk about… yes… *sustainability.*

The topic I was supposedly addressing was that of the possibilities of sustainability in the NGO sector and relates these to the experiences of ZIFF. In order to retain a freehearted, artistic essence, ZIFF is also re-imaging itself from annual beggar on a pilgrimage into gorgeous, single exotic person (female) seeking suitable larger organization in art, culture, creativity with which to share activities.

Some insights

First, there can be no authentic conclusions to this discussion unless the purpose and motives for which organizations are established are dealt with openly. Are we in it for the cause? The idea? The opportunity? The money?

Second: the epistemologies of development and development aid need to be laid bare if the topic is to gain any currency (no pun intended). Partners (donors) seemingly need NGOs to justify their own existence, especially to their taxpayers back home, and NGOs need donors for their existence. A symbiotic thing going on here, and heck, so far, it works. Or

Three: The very apparent need for institutional sustainability mechanisms even at a foundational level: at least the presence of an annual plan and a budget, in the midst of the very enthusiastic dreams, even if it is a subsidiary of a larger NGO based elsewhere. But the sustainability mechanisms include the need for a conversation in which there will be a tacit agreement that even if poverty eradication stops being trendy this year and the rehabilitation of cats becomes all the rage next year, the programmes established under poverty eradication should experience their fullest growth potential before everybody rushes to write up pieces on the viability of cats.

Four: There is need, perhaps, to expand the understanding of what an NGO is and what it can and should do. To engage more with the idea of social enterprises, and the donors/partners as providers of social capital for which some sort of returns ought to be expected.

Five: Particularly where creative energies are summoned by organizations to express a societal experience, growth depends significantly on the room given to imagination, a necessary but amorphous variable."

With those remarks, Yvonne Adhiambo rested her case.

Things to ponder about:

- Is it ethical for funders to require that implements of crucial / health programs be sustainable while even in rich nations sustainability is not achieved? Can we imagine sustainability at different levels?

- How can communities be more involved in program design and implementation? Would this help with continuity?

- Most organizations have no access to the private sector. How can they involve that sector?

XIII

A major component of EE initiative is the media. In a substantial number of cases, the media do not operate independently. Forces from government and the owners put pressure on editors and heads of departments to put aside content that may be seen to subvert certain interests. There is also self-censorship in which writers and editors interpret the potential implications of their media content and bottle it in fear of consequences. There are, of course, situations where the media over stretch themselves especially when involved in agenda setting or seeking great sales through sensitization of information.

At a Summit dinner in the centre of Nairobi, we sought to deliberate these events guided by a short presentation by Evan Mwangi then of the University of Nairobi with a response by Muthoni Wanyeki of Femnet. The two interventions are reproduced in their entirety. Whereas it may be viewed that issues of media regulation are extraneous to the subject of Entertainment-education, they are not. They are, in fact, at the centre of our pursuit to provide education in a non-threatening manners. Depending on the levels of tolerance for freedom of expression, media outlets could either facilitate or inhibit socially significant entertainment work.

Entertainment: Media Regulation vis-à-vis Democracy and Health

Evan Mwangi

Statement of Obvious Things: Aesthetics of Seriousness

"May I start by putting on a most serious face so that I can unashamedly repeat the obvious. The role of the media in development efforts and the nurturing of democracy in Africa cannot be gainsaid. The media are seen as important in informing, educating and entertaining the consumers of their products. A democratic system of governance would require, among other things, competition among individuals and organization and freedom of the press (Dahl 1989: 241; Diamond et al 1990:6-7; Hadenius 1993:35). Thus if a society is to consider itself to be democratic, it should allow the competition between media houses and the freedom of expression, which is considered the most important component of democracy (Gastil 1990: 25-26). This is because, to use Pnina Lahav words, press freedom as being "woven into the texture of modern democracy" (1995:339)

Media freedom is usually seen to mean the liberty to articulate political opinions, especially those that tend towards the radicals, against the grains of power and its various manifestations. We would like to widen this to encompass health issues that confront the nation. In which ways does the media facilitate or threaten health possibilities in the society? Should we allow any kind of entertainment to flow out of media outlets to prove that we are democratic? Are media that degrade women or pervert children to be allowed into Kenya communication space? How can they be regulated without reducing the democratic space that freedom of expression embodies?

We want to argue that measure should be put in place to ensure the media's role in promoting health and democracy and limiting the threats the media might pose to development. The subject of media regulation in Africa has preoccupied communication scholars for some time. The feeling has been that African media have been denied the right political and legal environment to operate freely and serve the society as meaningfully as they should. The focus in this discourse has largely been on the censorship of openly political news and programmes. We rarely think of the impact of regulation on entertainment and how that would affect democracy and other development facets of the society. Yet issue-based entertainment is the basis of African media. In folk media, for example, artistic expression is functional. Although art for art's sake may spring its head once in a while, it would be frowned upon and discouraged by the wider society. In Africa, thus, there is no amusement for amusement's sake, unless it is pathological enterprise.

Final Notes on the Postcolony

In this presentation in progress, I examine the role of media regulation on entertainment and how the regulation would affect larger policy instruments. We proceed from the Bakhtinian premise that entertainment is cardinal in regulating state power. We appropriate Russian theorist Mikhail Baktin concept of the carnivalesque to appreciate the place of entertainment industry and practices in the negotiation for wider and more profound political space. In the book *Rabelais and His World*, discusses how the popular culture in early modern Europe used comical flourishes to mock dictatorial tendencies and parody official ideas of society, history, destiny, as unalterable. For Bakhtin, carnivalesque entertainment "uses elements of parody, mimicry, bodily humour and grotesque display to achieve the ends of carnival, that is, to jostle 'from below' the univocal, elevated language of high art and decorous society". The festival of pleasure, that on the surface might appear irrational, became philosophical modes of expressing the societal hopes, fears and aspirations. Through extravagant juxtapositions, the grotesque mixing and confrontations of high and low, upper-class and lower-class, spiritual and material, young and old, male and female, daily identity and festive mask, serious conventions and their parodies, gloomy medieval time and joyous utopian visions. What we learn form Bakhtin is that spectacles and comic verbal compositions are an important aspect of the expression of the people's power against authoritarianism. Therefore, "the down to earth" media, which prioritize entertainment, would help the society deconstruct power and safeguard the democracy space.

While Bakhtin sees the carnivalesque to reside in the non-official realms of social practice by ordinary people, Achille Mbembe views the official discourse in Africa to be laced in a deep sense of the comical. The official/banal dichotomy is collapsed in such a way that African officials are themselves comedians in the public space leaders. For Mbembe, the timing and location is manipulated in such a way that the state extravagantly displays it magnificence as spectacle to the public (2001:104). It is no wonder that the postcolonial space in Africa is pervaded by comedy and self-display that entertainers pick up to criticize the fetishes with which the state comically exhibits itself to its subjects. It is no accident that state functions are pervaded by comical display or that comedians find their way into 'serious' political spaces. In Africa, the boundary between politics and the comical is quite porous.

Then, it would be in the interest of the nation - for it cannot avoid the comical - to structure entertainment into an issue-based enterprise in which its comical capital is utilized to highlight the problems of the postcolony and point to the nation's possible regeneration.

Liberalization: Libel and its Discontents

With a modicum of liberalization informing the Kenya environment towards the end of the last decade, entertainment industry has enjoyed greater space. There has been a sharp rise in the number of independent FM radio stations. The officials have also been parodied on TV programmes such as *Redykulas*, not to mention the greater freedom the cartoonist brushes have enjoyed to draw and satirize the powers that be. With the provision of the Internet, even the censored cartoons by *Gaddo* can be enjoyed online. In the face of unrelenting competition, older media houses that specialized as mouthpieces of the government have had to reposition themselves either by changing their news content or intensifying their entertainment package.

The fight between the state and ordinary folk produce more complicated carnival of self-display in which the state deconstructs its banality. For example, in 2002, Kenya Broadcasting Corporation, the national broadcaster, banned a song by *Gidi Gidi and Maji Maji* ostensibly because it had been appropriated by the Opposition as its anthem against the incumbent president Daniel Arap Moi in the presidential campaigns. The song, *I am Unbwogable*, may pass as any other irrational expression by drunken youths, but beneath it is a challenge to the state that it cannot subjugate Kenyans for ever. The song, popular in nightclubs perhaps because it seems so say absolutely nothing substantial, employs what Mbembe would call the aesthetics of abuse to challenge what the system, given to the carnivalesque imagination, saw as itself. The state is confronted, and feels itself challenged, by a simple song whose significance would ordinarily not go beyond the revelry of down-town night clubs:

What the hell are you looking for,
Can't a young Luo make money anymore?
Who are you?
What are you?
Who the hell do you think you are?
Get the hell out of my face...

The song does not only lament the stereotypes and ethnocentric marginalisation the state has helped to circulate, but it tells off the authority as well. The artist overthrows state power and assumes the power to dismiss the state "out of my face". He criticizes constant state policing in which the state is always "looking for" its subjects to expend its excesses on and limit their economic and democratic space.

The persona insists that he is *unbwogable*, indomitable, jesting in series of rhetorical questions that he is above the state control:

I am unbwogable!
I am unbeatable!
I am unsue-able!
I said, who can bwogo me?
Who can bwogo me?
Who can bwogo me?
Who can bwogo me?
I am unbwogable!

The word "unbwogable" is a coinage for the Dholuo word 'bwogo' (meaning beat, suppress, silence). Here it is anglicized through the use of the negative prefix "un" and the suffix "able". The new adjective variously means unbeatable, indomitable, insuppressible. The legal instrument of violence against entertainment are suggested when the persona claims that he cannot even be sued. Through neologism, expansion of vocabulary, the persona condemns social construction and unequivocally celebrates expansion of democracy and meaning.

By insisting that he cannot be repressed or intimidated by threats of legal suits the persona of *I am Unbwogable* suggests the repression of Kenya media through the courts. A litany of libel suits has dogged the Kenyan media industry in which the media houses have been forced to pay millions of shillings as damages. In the space of one year between 2001 and 2002, the Nation Media Group paid over 30 million Kenya shillings after being sued for libel. The Standard Group that owns *East African Standard* and Kenya Television Network has been ordered to pay a lawyer, 10 million Kenya shillings in a single libel award. The *People Daily* was ordered to pay Nicholas Biwott (a former cabinet Minister) Kshs. 20 million for a 1999 story on the Turkwell Hydro-Electric Power project, which his lawyers argued depicted him as a corrupt man. In December 2000, Biwott was awarded Kshs 30 million against British authors Dro Ian West and Chester Stern for implicating him in the murder of the former Foreign Affairs Minister Robert Ouko. Book Point, a leading outlet for entertainment and scholarly publications, was ordered to pay Kshs 10 million for selling the book that was allegedly libelous to Biwott. In such circumstances, the media can easily be forced into disabling self-censorship.

Pornography and the Freedom for those of us who Like it

While the official media maybe *bwogable,* the informal entertainment outlets offer greater potential for the expansion of democracy. Yet towards the end of 2001, the Kenyan government introduced various amendments to the constitution that would cripple the semi-formal media houses. The publishers are also required to submit copies of articles to the government, before circulation to the public. Media houses warned that this would introduce bureaucratic delays, which would hinder meeting strict deadlines.

It is important for health and democracy that bad media be controlled. With the media liberalization there is an influx of pornographic publication. Personal research indicates that a vendor sells about 100 copies of pornographic materials every week. While we are usually worried about children's consumption of bad media, it is the adult male who needs protection. The buyers are male readers above 35.

Incidentally, these buyers rarely ask for the publications if they are not on display as they would inquire about, say, mainstream newspapers and magazines if they are out of stock. This implies that if the pornographic magazines were not displayed, their buyers would not have the courage to ask for them. The consumers seem to be aware that they are consuming bad products. The problem might not really be in the publications, but the readers who might have some psychosexual problems. Yet the availability of the publications encourages their consumption. However, instead of banning them, we would submit that the readers should be sensitized against reading the materials. The committees in charge of media self-regulation should consider training the vendors on the ethics of Newspapers distribution so that the hapless vendors are not used to peddle sleaze. Mainstream media outlets could strictly contract vendors who do not stock pornography. This would enable only those who are proud of pornographic materials to peddle them openly without having to hide respectable newspapers.

At least good work is being done at the level of self-regulation. Despite accessibility of pornography on-line, there is a stricture is most cyber-cafés that clients should not open pornographic sites. The religious serve as regulating institutions. To widen the democratic space without veering into too-casual tastes, we should have more community radio stations broadcasting in local languages. *Kameme FM* is doing a good job in broadcasting in *Kikuyu* language. The fact that it is broadcasting in an African language, circumscribed by strict social codes, the station - even if it wanted - cannot broadcast the sleaze we are treated to by other FM radio stations which I suspect are modeled on something somebody listened to the last time they were in the West."

Ms. Muthoni Wanyeki, the Executive Director of the African Women's Development and Communication Network (FEMNET) responded to Mr. Mwangi's paper by giving a commentary of it in which she said

"Thank you for inviting me to speak this evening. I was asked to respond to Evan Mwangi's paper on the regulation of entertainment in Kenya and its impact on democracy, development and health. After three days of related discussions and debates and during a dinner such as this, I'm sure the topic does not entirely thrill you. So I ask you to bear with me—my task is not as hard as his, and I promise to take you through what I have to add fairly fast.

In the meantime, fill your glass with wine—it will help.

What are we Regulating and How?

Mwangi raises freedom of expression and competition as being two pre-requisites for democracy. I would agree with him that freedom of expression is indeed an essential pre-requisite although I feel that the idea that competition—in and of itself—is a debatable pre-requisite, for reasons, which I shall return to later. He goes further to note that freedom of expression has been primarily understood with respect to political opinion and posits that our understanding of freedom of expression should also incorporate our opinions on critical issues facing Africa, most notably health.

Again, I would agree with him, although I would go beyond our opinions on the whole range of human rights—civil and political rights, economic, social and cultural rights, the rights to development and peace as well as reproductive and sexual rights—all of which need to be understood from a gendered perspective.

When we take into account how those opinions are most typically shared, beyond one on one conversations and beyond gatherings such as this, we know that we are talking about the media and, more fundamentally, about the media's need for responsibility.

And yes, I am fully aware of the dread with which most African media practitioners and workers react to the combination of those words—media and responsibility—because they are words which have been repeatedly thrown into our faces when we raise those sticky questions about media and freedom).

How then are questions relating to media responsibility dealt with? The obvious answer is through regulation—the combination of constitutional provisions, laws and policies that seek to uphold the rights to freedom of expression and information, as well as to clarify, specify the practical means through which those rights will be both realized and limited. Which raises a further question: how is regulation understood?

Regulating Media Content

Mwangi's paper deals primarily with the regulation of content—the content of media right down to songs given airtime on the media (and I must say, I loved his analysis of what became the opposition's anthem during our last General Elections). He then poses the question as to whether or not the regulation of content is best achieved through legal means or the exercise of informed choice. Given our history (which is a history shared with many other African states), it is no doubt natural that we react rather badly to the idea of regulation through legal means. For our experience has shown us that regulation through legal means has almost inevitably meant the imposition of further and more devious limitations on our freedom of expression as realized through content on the print and broadcast media in particular.

By way of example, Mwangi raises the debilitating effect that Kenya's libel laws have had on the print media in Kenya—and we must remember here that libel only became the weapon of choice of the former establishment after Kenyans had waged a long and successful struggle to get sedition off the books. A range of similarly restrictive (if not outright oppressive) laws remain on the books, affecting film, literature, the performing arts, particularly theatre. These restrictions are not always brought to bear, as the popularity of plays now screened in bars across the country testifies to (for which we have playwrights such as Wahome Mutahi to thank, may he soon recover). However, the fact is that an urgent review of all such legislation is required.

Regulating the Environment within which the Media Operates

So, if regulation of media content through legal means has not always worked for us, would regulation through the exercise of informed choice work any better?

This, in turn, forces us to ask what guarantees choice? Mwangi's assumption is that competition does, and it does—but only to a certain extent. Certainly, as he points out, liberalization has led to the establishment of many new commercial media outlets, which has forced change upon the stodgy and repressed public media outlets—which still, however, function as state/ruling political party outlets.

But there is a difference between 'independent' media and 'pluralistic' media and change cannot only be quantitative—it must also be qualitative to truly be able to 'add value' to the concern of this gathering—how the entertainment media can better address the range of critical issues facing Africa—from conflict to HIV/AIDS.

Even a cursory examination shows that the public media are still the only media with national coverage. The commercial media are largely located in urban areas, that the ratio of local content relative to foreign content is low, that the quality of local coverage is equally low and so on and so forth.

This is not to say that there are not some legitimate reasons for this (including, for example, the refusal of the formal government to grant broadcast licenses and frequencies outside of the capital). Nor this is not to imply that efforts have not been made to improve the quality of local coverage and programming (Mwangi, for example, points to the development of cartoonists and the move of comedy acts from clubs to radio and television screens).

But this is to stress my points that independence does not necessarily lead to pluralism and quantity does not necessarily lead to quality. In short, competition as a strategy for increasing and improving local media content and supporting local media is not a sufficient strategy

Mwangi notes the need for 'down to earth media' and posits that the informal media might provide a better for the kind of entertainment media content that this gathering is concerned with (despite his making an interesting link between the upsurge in informal media and the availability of pornography).

However, what he does not adequately address as specific is what these 'down to earth' and informal media are. I would submit that they are community media (although not in the sense that he has defined them)—that is media that are by, for and about their audiences and that are owned, managed and produced by those audiences

I therefore support here the demands that have been made over the past decade or so for regulation that recognizes the distinct differences between and the specific needs of public, commercial and community media. Such regulation would include a re-definition of the public media so that it can function as genuinely public media and provide clearly distinct licensing obligations on public, commercial and community media, with high quotas for local content being imposed on public and community media and specific frequency blocks being reserved for community media

There is, unfortunately (for me, not for you) no time to go into the specifics (although they are available and have just been availed to our Chief Guest following years of back and forth between the regulator and the two Ministries concerned).

So in conclusion, I would simply reiterate that regulation is about much more than media content. It is about determining the kind of media environment that we wish to have so as to ensure media pluralism in the future. For media pluralism is what will guarantee us choice. Choice as media producers about what to produce, how to fund its production and where to place it to ensure it reaches whom it is meant to reach.

And to choice as media consumers as to whether or not we want to listen to or watch programmes bemoaning the state of our individual hearts and pockets or programmes that reflect who we truly are, here in Africa, in all of our complexity."

Things to ponder about:

- All of us whether performers, media, artist or donors should mainstream gender in our areas of work and should avoid criminalizing women for example in the issue of feminization of HIV.

- We should consciously and deliberately mainstream and lobby gender issues.

- We should highlight the issues of persons with disabilities as well as harness young talent and create opportunities for them.

- Donors and artists should engage in dialogue once projects acquire funding in order to avoid tension and achieve sustainability.

- Other ways of fundraising and mobilizing resources should be explored rather than artists relying entirely on donors.

- Relationships with media owners and involving them in the work of artists should be explored.

- The capacities of our collaborators should be built to sensitize them particularly in the area of gender.

XIV

The Summit was inspirational in multiple ways and writers put their feelings on paper. Below, a poet celebrates the meeting of artists and cultural scholars.

'A Praise Song for You'

Let me sing you a praise song
My sister my brother,
Telling of your long journey
From the West to the East;
From the South to the North;
From the North to South;
Telling how we met in Nairobi
For the soap summit
Two thousand and three.

Let me sing a praise song
My sister, my brother,
Let me celebrate our oneness.
Let me dance for you
And tantalize you
With African rhythm
With my vibrancy!
Let me beat my drum
In your honor
My sister, my brother;
Let the African beat
Make your heart throb
With the joy of life!
Let me paint of your portrait
And capture the beauty

Of your eyes,
Capture the beauty
Of your smile,
Capture the beauty
Of your being!

Let me sing you a praise song
My sister, my brother,
Let me celebrate oneness.
Let my praise song tell
How we've eaten together,
How we've listened to each other,
How we've questioned
How we've answered,
Let my praise song tell
How we've reached conclusions
And in conclusions
In our deliberations.
Let my praise song tell
How we've probed our hearts,
How we've searched our minds,
And looked deep within our hearts
For answers hidden there.
Let my praise song tell
How we've examined each other
Surreptitiously;
How we've speculated about origins
Surreptitiously;
Wondered who we really are,
Wondered what we're about.

Let me sing a praise song
My sister, my brother,
Let me sing celebrate our oneness.
Let my praise song remind you
Of the story of the tortoise
Whose shell was shattered

And remains scarred forever,
But let my song tell
That it is this shattering
That makes the tortoise
A true survivor
Like our Continent Africa.
Let my praise song tell
That the scars of yesterday's
Misunderstanding
And misconceptions
Are not indelible;
Let my praise song tell
That these scars
Are but a mosaic of strength-
Yours and mine.
Let the praise song tell
How we've listened carefully
To the story of a mirror
In which we saw ourselves.
Let my praise song tell
Of another mirror- splendid-
Which reproduces our faces
To infinity-
Which creates a beautiful
Mosaic of our oneness.
Let me beat my drum
In your honor
My sister my brother,
Let its African beat
Celebrate the goodness
Of our shared humanity!

by Elizabeth Orchardson-Mazrui

XV

Conclusion

Thus far, we have explored a number of thought provoking reflection by a people involved in Entertainment-Education work. Through their own voices, they have shown us that despite the gains made so far in linking culture, entertainment and health much more needs to be done. There is need for more research based interventions that are culturally sensitive. There are calls for more networking and collaboration. And Africa ought to be seen not just as a place where problems are found but more so where solutions could be found. Important work is being undertaken in the continent but due to constraints of documentation, these efforts go unregistered. The Nairobi event was, therefore, important because it created a space for people in the Entertainment-Education industry an opportunity to share their approaches and thoughts. At the end of the meeting, a declaration on the way forward was shared. It is reproduced below:

Way Forward/Declaration

Nairobi Declaration - June 2003

The countries of Africa are bound together by the urgent and unique challenges of the twenty-first century. Africans must stop the HIV/AIDS pandemic without forgetting the humanity of those infected and affected by HIV/ AIDS. Africans must make reproductive health information and services available to all, while remembering that their use must be voluntary. Africans must achieve social and political development grounded in our unique and diverse cultures.

We are uncompromisingly optimistic about the future of Africa and its people in all their diversity and the vital role issue-based entertainment (commonly referred to as entertainment-education, enter-educate, and edutainment) must play in meeting these challenges. Our optimism is grounded in the 20 years of demonstrated success with issue-based entertainment in many countries throughout the continent. Twenty years of experience has created a skilled and diverse pool of writers, actors, producers, and researchers who are already engaged in making a better Africa. Twenty years of demonstrated success has created a pool of financial supporters, government agencies, and non-governmental agencies that are committed to providing the resources, support and the structure to enable our work.

Our vision for the next 20 years is to build on this past success by spreading the issue- based entertainment methodology to all countries in Africa. We, the issue- based entertainment community, meeting at the 2003 Nairobi Soap Summit on Making Entertainment Useful, June 3 to 7, 2003, commit ourselves to the advancement of issue -based entertainment on the continent of Africa and globally.

Our commitment includes the following positions and actionable steps:

1. To use proven issue- based entertainment methodologies of production and implementation;

2. To use the creative energies of our artists to serve our educational goals;

3. To make the educational issues of our programs relevant and accessible to all populations;

4. To make our programs as entertaining as possible so that they will draw the largest possible audience without compromising the ethical frameworks that guide our programs;

5. To build our programs on the oral traditions of African culture;

6. To respect the cultures of all our audiences;

7. To understand that the process of behavior change is slow and that our commitment must be sustained over time;

8.   To adhere to the highest standards of program production possible;

9.   To remain connected to our colleagues worldwide for a continuous exchange of ideas;

10. To build the capacity of our writers, actors, producers and researchers so that the pool of talent will grow and improve;

11. To explore the use of various media and to use multiple media to reinforce our educational themes and reach the largest possible audience;

12. To collaborate with academic scholars in communication and public health so that our interventions will be studied and disseminated;

13. To create lasting networks and professional institutions engaged in issue-based education for sustainability;

14. To collaborate with our colleagues regionally to share our successes and our experiences;

15. To reach out to the owners of the media to provide the idea that social and commercial interests can be both met through issue-based entertainment;

16. To develop and study the use of grassroots and alternative broadcast methodologies (community radio, short wave and digital rebroadcast platforms.)

17. To collaborate with cultural, social and, political icons and opinion leaders to disseminate information for social change;

18. To generate local resources as a strategy to achieving sustainability;

19. To call upon the donor community to work as equal partners in generating an agenda for issue-based entertainment programs,

striking a balance between donor interests, audience needs, and creative outputs;

20. To document and disseminate the processes and best practices of practitioners within the continent;

21. To advocate the use of issue-based entertainment and related communication strategies as an integral part of global health strategies at the local, national and international levels.

Next Actionable Steps:

1. We call for hosting an entertainment-education soap summit at least once every two years on the African continent to share experiences and best practices, to foster networking and collaborations, and to generate advocacy for issue-based entertainment among donors, media production houses, governments and the general public.

2. We call for instituting a set of awards to recognize African excellence in issue-based entertainment production and implementation. Guidelines for the open competition, award categorizes, and a small consultative group will develop selection process.

References

Ajayi, A. A. Eta al. (1991) " Adolescent sexuality and Fertility in Kenya: A Survey of Knowledge, Preceptions, and Attitudes" Studies in Family Planning Vol. 22 No. 4.

Bakhtin, Mikhail (1986). *Speech Genres and Other Late Essays* ed. Emerson and M. Holquist, trans. V.W. McGee. Austin: University of Texas Press.

Bandura, A. (1977) *Social learning theory*. Englewood Cliffs. N.J. Prentice-Hall.

Bandura, A. (1997) *Self-efficacy: The exercise of control*. New York: Freeman.

Bankole, A., Rodriguez, C., & Westoff, C.F. (1996). *Mass Media Messages and Reproductive Behavior in Nigeria*. Journal of Bioscience, 28, 227-239.

Barker, Gary Knaul and Susan Rich (1992) "Influences on adolescent sexuality in Nigeria and Kenya: Findings from recent focus-group discussions." *Studies in Family Planning* 23(3): 199-210.

Bentley, Eric (1965) *The Life of Drama*. London: Menthuen and Co.Ltd.

Brooke, Pamela (1995) *Communication through Story Characters*. Institute for International Research: University Press of America.

Crook, Tim (1999) *Radio Drama: Theory and Practice*. New York, Routledge.

Elber, Lynn (2000) *Population group's soap operas focus on life lessons, not lust*. The Chicago Tribune: Associated Press

Fairclough, Norman, (1992). *Discourse and Social Change*. Cambridge: Polity Press.

Government of Kenya. (1995) *The National Implementation Plan*: Kenya Family Planning Programme 1995-2000.

Government of Kenya. (1997) *Reproductive Health/Family Planning Policy Guidelines and Standards for Service Providers.* Ministry of Health, Nairobi.

Jackson, Hellen (2002) *AIDS Africa: Continent in Crisis.* Harare, SAfAIDS.

Jakarta Declaration on Leading Health Promotion into the 21st Century. World Health Organization, Geneva, 1997.

Kenya Demographic Health Survey (1993) NCPD-Central Bureau of Statistics (CBS) Office of the President and Ministry of Planning.

Kenya Demographic Health Survey (1998, 2003).

Khasiani & Njiro (1993). *The Women's Movement,* Nairobi, Association of African Women for Research and Development (AAWORD-Kenya).

Khasiani, S.A. (1985) *"Adolescent Fertility in Kenya with Special Reference to High School Teenage Pregnancy and Childbearing"* PRSI-University of Nairobi.

Kibwana, Kivutha (Ed.). (1995) Women and Autonomy in Kenya: Policy and Legal Framework, Claripress, Nairobi.

Kimani Njogu (2001) *Discourse and Serial Drama in the Promotion of Health in Kenya*: Kiswahili: A Tool for Development. Department of Kiswahili and Other African Languages and CHAKITA, Moi University Press.

Kimani Njogu (2004) *Reading Poetry as Dialogue.*, Nairobi, Jomo Kenyatta Foundation.

Kiragu K.and Zabin L.S. . 1992 *"The Correlates of Premarital Sexual Activity Among In-School Adolescents in Nakuru District, Kenya."* A Paper presented at the first inter-Africa Conference on Adolescents Nairobi Kenya, March 24-27, 1992.

Kiragu, K. 1991 " The Correlates of Sexual and Contraceptive Behaviour Among School Adolescents in Kenya" PhD. Thesis The JHU: Baltimore.

Lema, V.M. & Mulandi T. N. (1992). *"Knowledge and Attitudes Related to AIDS and HIV Infection among Adolescents in Nairobi:"* Center for the Study of Adolescents.

Lema V.M et al (1989) *"Epidemiology of Abortion in Kenya"* The Centre for the Study of Adolescence in Kenya. Nairobi.

Lema, V.M. (1987) *" Sexual Knowledge and Behaviour and Its Relationship to Contraceptive Knowledge, Attitudes, and Practice Among Adolescent Secondary School Girls in Nairobi."*

Lema. V.M (1989) *"Factors Associated with Adolescent Sexuality Among Secondary School Girls in Nairobi, Kenya."* Paper Presented at the 14th Annual Scientific Conference of the Kenya Obsterical and Gynaecological Society held on 22nd-24th February.

Marangu, J.M 1985. *"Incidence of Induced Abortion in Kenyatta National Hospital"* Faculty of Nursing - College of Health Profession, University of Nairobi.

Mazrui, Alamin, et. al, (1988)"A Formative Survey of *'Ushikwapo Shikamana,"* June – October. Prepared for NCPD, Nairobi.

Nariman, Heidi Noel (1993) *Soap Operas for Social Change: Toward a Methodology for Entertainment-Education Television.* Westport, CT: Praeger.

National Population Advocacy and IEC Strategy for Sustainable Development 1996-2010 (June 1996) NCPD, Nairobi.

National Research Council. 1993. *"Population Dynamics of Kenya",* National Academy Press: Washington D.C.

Nduati, Ruth & Wambui Kiai. 1993. *Communicating with Adolescents on HIV/AIDS in East and Southern Africa.* IDRC.

Njau, P. W. 1992. *"Tradtional sex Education"* Paper presented at the First Inter-African Conference on adolescent Health heald at Safari Park Hotel, Nairobi.

Ochillo, P.O. 1990. "A Summative Survey of *Ushikwapo Shikamana* Radio Soap Opera". Prepared for the National Council on Population and Development.

Okemwa, P. F. (1993). "The Place and Role of Women in the SDA Church in Kenya" Unpublished M.A. thesis, Kenyatta university.

Okumu, Y. M and Chege N.I 1994. *"Female Adolescent Health and Sexuality in Kenyan secondary Schools. A Survey Report"* AMREF: Nairobi.

POFLEP (Population/Family Life Education Programme) (1994) *Perceptions of Family Welfare, Family Planning and AIDS among Selected Cultural Clusters in Tanzania.* Dar es Salaam: Ministry of Community Development, Women Affairs, and Children. Report to the United Nations Population Fund.

Rogers, Everett M., Peter Vaughan, Ramadhan M.A. Swalehe, Nagesh Rao, Peer Svenkerud, Suruchi Sood, and Krista L. Alford. (1997) *Effects of an Entertainment-Education Radio Soap Opera on Family Planning and HIV/AIDS Prevention Behaviour in Tanzania.* Albuquerque and Arusha, Tanzania: University of New Mexico, Department of Communication and Journalism, and Population/Family Life Education Programme.

Rogo K. & Njau. 1994. *"Newspaper Articles on Family Life Education/Sex Education in Kenya."* Centre for the Study of Adolescence: Nairobi.

Rogo, K. 1993. *"Analysis and Documentation of Research on Adolescent Sexuality and Unsafe Abortion"* Centre for the Study of Adolescence: Nairobi.

Rogo, Khama. 1995. *"Research Findings on Women and Health in Kenya: Developing an Action Agenda."* In Kivutha Kibwana *Women and Autonomy in Kenya: Policy and Legal Framework*, Claripress, Nairobi.

Said, Edward W. (1993) *Culture and Imperialism.* New York, Vintage Books.

Singhal, Arvind and Everett M. Rogers (1999) *Entertainment-Education: A Communication Strategy for Social Change*. Mahwah, NJ: Lawrence Erlbaum Associates.

The Children of Africa Confront AIDS (2003) (edited by Arvind Singhal and W. Stephen Howard). Ohio University Research in International Studies Africa series No. 80, Ohio University Press

Westoff, C. F. & Rodriguez, C. (1995). *The Mass Media and Family Planning in Kenya*. International Family Planning Perspectives 21, 1.

www.ingramcontent.com/pod-product-compliance
Lightning Source LLC
Chambersburg PA
CBHW021902020426
42334CB00013B/436